Embodied Healing

The Complete Body-Based Guide to Nervous System Reset and Trauma Recovery

Harold Amon MacKay

Copyright © 2025 by Harold Amon MacKay

All rights reserved. No part of this publication may be reproduced, distributed, or transmitted in any form or by any means, including photocopying, recording, or other electronic or mechanical methods, without the prior written permission of the publisher, except in the case of brief quotations embodied in critical reviews and certain other noncommercial uses permitted by copyright law.

Isohan Publishing

First Edition: 2025

ISBN: 978-1-7641941-7-4

This book is for educational and informational purposes only and is not intended as medical, psychological, or therapeutic advice. The content provided herein does not constitute professional medical advice, diagnosis, or treatment. Always seek the advice of your physician, mental health professional, or other qualified healthcare provider with any questions you may have regarding a medical condition, mental health concern, or trauma-related symptoms.

The somatic exercises, techniques, and practices described in this book are general in nature and may not be appropriate for everyone. Do not disregard professional medical advice or delay seeking professional help because of something you have read in this book. If you are experiencing thoughts of self-harm, suicide, or harm to others, please seek immediate professional help or contact emergency services.

The names and scenarios depicted in this book are purely for illustrative purposes only. Any resemblance to actual persons, living or dead, or actual events is purely coincidental. Case studies and examples have been created to demonstrate concepts and techniques and do not represent real individuals or their experiences.

While the practices and information contained in this book are based on established therapeutic approaches and research, no specific outcomes or results are guaranteed. Healing is a highly individual process, and what works for one person may not work for another.

Table of Contents

Chapter 1: Your Body's Wisdom 1
   What is Somatic Therapy 1
   The Mind-Body Connection Explained 2
   How Trauma Lives in the Body 3
   Your Healing Journey Roadmap.. 4
   Initial Self-Assessment: Body Awareness Inventory........... 5
   Exercise 1.1: Basic Body Scan Meditation 6
   Exercise 1.2: Identifying Your Body's Stress Signals 7
   Exercise 1.3: Creating Your Healing Intention.................... 8
   Worksheet: Personal Trauma Impact Map........................ 10

Chapter 2: Building Your Foundation............................... 13
   Understanding Your Window of Tolerance...................... 13
   Creating Internal and External Safety 14
   The Power of Co-regulation.. 16
   When to Seek Professional Support................................... 17
   Exercise 2.1: Establishing Your Safe Space Visualization 19
   Exercise 2.2: Grounding Through the Five Senses........... 20
   Exercise 2.3: Building Your Resource Library 21
   Worksheet: Safety Planning Template............................... 23

Chapter 3: Developing Body Literacy............................... 26
   Sensation vs. Emotion vs. Thought..................................... 26
   The SIBAM Model 28
   Tracking Activation and Deactivation 30
   Understanding Your Nervous System States 32

Exercise 3.1: Sensation Vocabulary Building 34
Exercise 3.2: Daily Sensation Tracking Practice 36
Exercise 3.3: Pendulation - Riding the Waves................ 38
Exercise 3.4: Noticing Without Changing 40
Worksheet: Personal Sensation Dictionary...................... 41
Building Your Somatic Foundation................................ 43

Chapter 4: Conscious Breathing for Healing 45
The Science of Breathwork and Trauma 45
Different Breathing Patterns and Their Effects................ 47
Breath as a Bridge Between Voluntary and Involuntary .. 48
Exercise 4.1: Three-Dimensional Breathing..................... 50
Exercise 4.2: Coherent Breathing (5-5 Rhythm) 51
Exercise 4.3: The Physiological Sigh 53
Exercise 4.4: Breath for Activation and Calming............. 54
Exercise 4.5: Voo Breath for Vagus Nerve...................... 56
Worksheet: Personal Breath Practice Plan...................... 58
The Breathing Foundation 60

Chapter 5: Releasing Trauma Through Motion 62
Why Movement Heals 62
The Difference Between Exercise and Therapeutic Movement 64
Finding Your Movement Style 65
Exercise 5.1: Gentle Shaking for Discharge 67
Exercise 5.2: Spontaneous Movement Exploration 69
Exercise 5.3: Wall Push-Offs for Boundary Work 71
Exercise 5.4: Figure-8 Flowing Movements..................... 73
Exercise 5.5: Dance Your Emotions................................. 74

Exercise 5.6: Tension and Release Sequences 76
Worksheet: Movement Comfort Zone Map 78
Moving Into Wholeness 80

Chapter 6: Reclaiming Your Physical Self 82
The Importance of Touch in Healing 82
Self-Touch as a Therapeutic Tool 84
Boundary Work Through the Body 85
Exercise 6.1: Self-Holding Practices 86
Exercise 6.2: Butterfly Hug for Self-Soothing 88
Exercise 6.3: Body Boundary Visualization 90
Exercise 6.4: Progressive Muscle Relaxation 2.0 92
Exercise 6.5: Partner Exercises for Co-Regulation (Optional) 94
Worksheet: Boundary Assessment and Goals 96
Reclaiming Your Physical Self 99

Chapter 7: Healing Through Resonance 101
How Sound Affects the Nervous System 101
Using Your Voice for Healing 103
Vibrational Therapy Basics 104
Exercise 7.1: Humming for Vagus Nerve Activation 106
Exercise 7.2: Toning for Emotional Release 107
Exercise 7.3: Sound Bath Creation 109
Exercise 7.4: Chanting and Repetition 111
Exercise 7.5: Music for Nervous System Regulation 113
Worksheet: Personal Sound Healing Playlist 115
Resonating with Healing 118

Chapter 8: Integration Practices 120

Combining Modalities for Deeper Healing................... 120
Creating Your Personal Practice 122
Working with Resistance and Obstacles 123
Exercise 8.1: Morning Somatic Ritual........................... 124
Exercise 8.2: Evening Discharge Practice 126
Exercise 8.3: SOS Emergency Regulation Sequence 128
Exercise 8.4: Weekly Integration Session..................... 130
Exercise 8.5: Body-Based Problem Solving.................. 132
Worksheet: Personalized Practice Schedule 134
Weaving the Threads of Healing 136

Chapter 9: Targeted Healing Approaches..................... 138
Developmental Trauma Adaptations 138
Shock Trauma Responses 140
Complex PTSD Considerations 141
Cultural and Collective Trauma..................................... 143
Exercise 9.1: Inner Child Body Dialogue 145
Exercise 9.2: Releasing Hypervigilance Patterns 147
Exercise 9.3: Reconnecting After Dissociation 150
Exercise 9.4: Anger Discharge Sequences.................... 152
Exercise 9.5: Grief Movement Rituals........................... 154
Worksheet: Trauma Pattern Identification..................... 156
Addressing Your Unique Healing Path.......................... 159

Chapter 10: Somatic Healing with Others..................... 161
The Neurobiology of Connection 161
Co-regulation vs. Self-regulation................................... 163
Healing Attachment Through the Body 164

Exercise 10.1: Eye Contact Titration 166

Exercise 10.2: Synchronized Breathing 169

Exercise 10.3: Safe Touch Exploration........................... 171

Exercise 10.4: Conflict Resolution Through Body Awareness 173

Worksheet: Relationship Somatic Patterns 176

The Heart of Healing.. 179

Chapter 11: Living Somatically 180

Making Somatic Awareness a Lifestyle......................... 180

Preventing Re-traumatization 182

Continued Growth and Development 183

Exercise 11.1: Daily Life Movement Practices 185

Exercise 11.2: Workplace Regulation Techniques 187

Exercise 11.3: Somatic Parenting Basics 190

Exercise 11.4: Community and Collective Healing........ 193

Final Assessment: Progress Celebration 196

Worksheet: Future Vision and Goals 198

Your Somatic Life Awaits 201

Chapter 12: Your Ongoing Journey - Resources and Next Steps 204

When and How to Find a Somatic Therapist 204

Recommended Training Programs................................. 207

Building Your Support Network.................................... 209

Continuing Education Options....................................... 211

Creating Healing Communities...................................... 213

Professional Directory Guide... 215

Your Continued Journey 218

Resources for Continued Learning **219**
References **222**

Chapter 1: Your Body's Wisdom

The human body speaks a language older than words—a language of sensation, movement, and cellular memory that holds the keys to healing trauma. This ancient wisdom operates below the threshold of conscious thought, yet it remains accessible to those who learn its vocabulary. Modern neuroscience has finally caught up with what indigenous healers have known for millennia: the body remembers everything, and within that memory lies both our wounds and our capacity for restoration.

Somatic therapy represents a paradigm shift in how we approach healing. Rather than focusing solely on cognitive processes or emotional expression, this approach recognizes that trauma leaves its mark in the tissues, nervous system, and movement patterns of the body (1). The word "somatic" derives from the Greek "soma," meaning the living body in its wholeness—not just the physical form, but the entire organism as an integrated system of sensation, movement, and awareness.

What is Somatic Therapy

Somatic therapy operates on a fundamental premise: the body possesses an innate capacity for self-regulation and healing when given the proper conditions and support. This approach views symptoms not as pathology to be eliminated, but as adaptive responses that once served a protective function (2). The goal becomes helping the nervous system complete interrupted defensive responses and return to a state of dynamic equilibrium.

Consider the case of Maria, a 34-year-old teacher who came to therapy following a car accident. While she had no serious physical injuries, she found herself unable to drive, experiencing panic attacks, and feeling disconnected from her body. Traditional talk therapy helped her understand her anxiety cognitively, but her nervous system remained locked in a state of hyperarousal. Through somatic work, Maria learned to track the sensations in her body—the tightness in her chest, the clenching in her jaw, the urge to flee. Gradually, she began to notice moments when her system naturally moved toward calm. By following these organic impulses toward regulation, her nervous system slowly released the trapped survival energy from the accident.

The therapeutic process involved no dramatic breakthroughs or forced emotional releases. Instead, Maria learned to be present with her body's responses, to track sensation without immediately trying to change it, and to support her nervous system's natural movement toward balance. Over several months, her symptoms gradually resolved as her body completed the defensive responses that had been interrupted during the trauma.

The Mind-Body Connection Explained

The artificial separation between mind and body represents one of the most limiting beliefs in modern healthcare. Neuroscientist Antonio Damasio's research demonstrates that emotion and feeling emerge from bodily states, not the other way around (3). The brain constantly receives input from internal organs, muscles, and sensory systems, creating what researchers call "interoception"—the felt sense of the body's internal state.

This connection operates through multiple pathways. The vagus nerve, the longest cranial nerve, carries information between the brain and major organs, influencing heart rate, digestion, and immune function. The autonomic nervous system responds to environmental cues within milliseconds, preparing the body for action before conscious awareness occurs. Neural networks throughout the gut contain more neurons than the spinal cord, earning recognition as the "second brain" (4).

James, a combat veteran, experienced this mind-body connection firsthand. After multiple deployments, he struggled with insomnia, digestive issues, and emotional numbness. His body remained vigilant even in safe environments, scanning for threats that weren't present. Traditional approaches focused on changing his thoughts about safety, but his nervous system continued operating from survival mode.

Through somatic work, James learned to recognize the subtle signs of activation in his body—the slight tension in his shoulders, the quickening of his breath, the narrowing of his visual field. He practiced simple exercises like feeling his feet on the ground and noticing his breathing pattern. Gradually, his nervous system began to distinguish between past danger and present safety. His sleep improved, his digestion normalized, and he regained access to a fuller range of emotions.

How Trauma Lives in the Body

Trauma occurs when an event overwhelms the nervous system's capacity to cope, leaving the individual feeling helpless and unable to respond effectively (5). The body's natural defense mechanisms—fight, flight, or freeze—become activated but cannot complete their protective function. This incomplete response creates what somatic practitioners call "trapped survival energy."

Dr. Bessel van der Kolk's groundbreaking research reveals that trauma fundamentally alters brain structure and function (6). The amygdala, responsible for threat detection, becomes hyperactive. The prefrontal cortex, governing rational thought and planning, shows decreased activity. Most significantly, the areas of the brain responsible for integrating sensory experience become disrupted, leaving individuals feeling disconnected from their bodies.

This disconnection serves as a protective mechanism initially but becomes problematic over time. Sarah, a survivor of childhood abuse, described feeling like she was "living from the neck up." She excelled academically and professionally but struggled with intimate relationships and self-care. Her body felt foreign to her, and she experienced frequent illness despite medical tests showing nothing wrong.

Through somatic therapy, Sarah gradually learned to inhabit her body again. She started with simple practices like noticing her breathing and feeling her feet on the floor. Initially, even these basic exercises triggered anxiety, but her therapist guided her to notice and respect these responses rather than override them. Over time, Sarah developed what somatic practitioners call "embodied presence"—the ability to be aware of physical sensations without becoming overwhelmed by them.

The process wasn't linear. Some days Sarah felt more connected to her body; others, she retreated into familiar patterns of disconnection. Her therapist helped her understand this as a natural part of healing rather than failure. Gradually, Sarah's capacity for presence expanded, and she began experiencing emotions as physical sensations rather than overwhelming floods. Her relationships deepened as she became more available to connection with others.

Your Healing Journey Roadmap

Somatic healing follows a non-linear path that honors the body's own timing and wisdom. Unlike cognitive approaches that focus on understanding and insight, somatic work emphasizes direct experience and gradual capacity building. The process typically involves three phases: stabilization, integration, and expansion (7).

The stabilization phase focuses on developing resources and increasing tolerance for sensation. Clients learn to track their internal experience, identify signs of activation and calm, and develop practices that support nervous system regulation. This phase may last weeks, months, or longer, depending on individual history and circumstances.

Integration involves slowly working with activation while maintaining connection to resources. Rather than flooding clients with intense sensation or emotion, the approach emphasizes titration—working with small amounts of activation at a time. This allows the nervous system to process and integrate experience without becoming overwhelmed.

The expansion phase focuses on building capacity for fuller engagement with life. Clients develop greater tolerance for both activation and calm, expanded emotional range, and improved relational capacity. The work becomes less about symptom management and more about supporting ongoing growth and resilience.

Initial Self-Assessment: Body Awareness Inventory

Before beginning formal exercises, take time to assess your current relationship with your body. This inventory provides a baseline for tracking progress and identifying areas that need particular attention.

Find a comfortable seated position and close your eyes. Begin by simply noticing your body as a whole. What draws your attention first? Some people immediately notice areas of tension or discomfort; others may feel relatively calm. Neither response is better than the other—simply observe what's present for you right now.

Now systematically scan through different areas of your body. Start with your head and face. Notice the muscles around your eyes, jaw, and forehead. Move down to your neck and shoulders.

What do you find there? Continue through your arms, chest, upper back, abdomen, lower back, hips, legs, and feet.

As you scan, notice the quality of sensation in each area. Some regions may feel tense, others relaxed. You might notice temperature, pressure, tingling, or numbness. Some areas may feel very present and alive, while others seem difficult to sense at all. Again, simply observe without trying to change anything.

Pay attention to your breathing throughout this process. Does it change as you focus on different body parts? Does it feel natural and easy, or restricted in some way?

Finally, notice your overall sense of being in your body. Do you feel connected and present, or somewhat detached? Can you sense your body's boundaries—where you end and the external world begins?

This inventory isn't about finding problems to fix but rather developing the skill of interoception—the ability to sense your internal state. Like any skill, it improves with practice.

Exercise 1.1: Basic Body Scan Meditation

This foundational practice develops body awareness and begins training the nervous system to tolerate sensation without immediately moving into reaction.

Sit or lie down in a comfortable position where you won't be disturbed for 15-20 minutes. Close your eyes or soften your gaze downward. Begin by noticing three things you can hear in your environment. This helps orient your nervous system to the present moment.

Now bring your attention to your breathing. Don't try to change it—simply notice the natural rhythm of inhalation and exhalation. If your mind wanders, gently return attention to your breath.

Starting at the top of your head, slowly move your attention through different parts of your body. Spend 30-60 seconds with each area, simply noticing whatever sensations are present. You might feel warmth, coolness, tingling, pressure, tension, or nothing at all. Each response is perfectly fine.

Move through your forehead, eyes, cheeks, jaw, and neck. Notice your shoulders, arms, and hands. Bring attention to your chest and upper back, feeling your ribcage expand and contract with each breath. Continue to your abdomen, lower back, hips, thighs, knees, calves, and feet.

If you encounter areas that feel numb or difficult to sense, don't force awareness. Simply acknowledge the absence of sensation and move on. Sometimes numbness is the nervous system's way of protecting against overwhelming input.

Similarly, if you notice areas of intense sensation or discomfort, avoid the urge to immediately change or fix them. Practice simply being present with whatever you find. If sensation becomes too intense, shift your attention to an area that feels more neutral or comfortable.

Complete the scan by sensing your body as a whole. Notice the general quality of aliveness or energy in your system. End by returning to awareness of your breathing and slowly opening your eyes.

Exercise 1.2: Identifying Your Body's Stress Signals

Your body provides constant feedback about your internal state, but many people have learned to ignore or override these signals. This exercise helps you recognize your personal stress indicators so you can respond before overwhelm occurs.

Over the next week, practice checking in with your body several times throughout the day. Set reminders on your phone or use natural transition points like before meals or when entering your car. Each check-in takes only 30-60 seconds.

During each check-in, ask yourself: "What is my body telling me right now?" Notice physical sensations, but also observe:

- Breathing pattern: Is it shallow or deep? Fast or slow? Smooth or irregular?
- Muscle tension: Where do you hold stress in your body? Common areas include shoulders, jaw, stomach, and lower back.
- Energy level: Do you feel energized, depleted, or somewhere in between?
- Overall nervous system state: Do you feel calm, agitated, spacey, or hyperalert?

Pay particular attention to these signals during stressful situations. Notice what happens in your body when you're running late, dealing with conflict, or facing deadlines. Does your breathing change? Do certain muscles tighten? Does your temperature shift?

Also observe your stress signals in different environments. How does your body respond in crowded spaces versus quiet ones? At work versus at home? With certain people versus others?

Keep notes about these observations. After a week, review your findings. You'll likely notice patterns in how your body responds to different types of stress. This awareness becomes the foundation for developing personalized regulation strategies.

Exercise 1.3: Creating Your Healing Intention

Intention setting in somatic work differs from goal setting in cognitive approaches. Rather than focusing on eliminating symptoms or achieving specific outcomes, somatic intentions emphasize process and capacity building.

Begin by settling into your body using the body scan technique from Exercise 1.1. When you feel present and grounded, bring to mind your desire for healing. What called you to this work? What do you hope to develop or restore?

Notice how this intention feels in your body. Does it create expansion or contraction? Excitement or anxiety? Energy or fatigue? These bodily responses provide important information about the authenticity and accessibility of your intention.

If your initial intention creates tension or overwhelm in your body, consider modifying it. Instead of "I want to heal all my trauma," you might say "I want to develop a kinder relationship with my body." Instead of "I want to eliminate anxiety," try "I want to increase my capacity to be present with difficult emotions."

Effective somatic intentions often include:

- Building capacity rather than eliminating problems
- Developing relationship with your body rather than controlling it
- Increasing tolerance for sensation and emotion
- Expanding your window of tolerance for activation and calm
- Learning to trust your body's wisdom

Write your intention down and place it somewhere you'll see it regularly. Return to it periodically throughout your healing process, noticing how it may shift and change as you grow.

Worksheet: Personal Trauma Impact Map

This worksheet helps you identify how trauma has affected different areas of your life and body. Complete it at your own pace, taking breaks as needed. If any section feels too activating, skip it and return later.

Physical Symptoms:

- What physical symptoms do you experience regularly?
- Which parts of your body hold the most tension or discomfort?
- How has trauma affected your sleep, appetite, or energy levels?
- What physical activities or movements feel difficult or triggering?

Emotional Patterns:

- What emotions do you experience most frequently?
- Which emotions feel difficult to access or express?
- How do you typically cope with overwhelming feelings?
- What emotional patterns would you like to change?

Relationships:

- How has trauma affected your ability to trust others?
- What challenges do you experience in intimate relationships?
- How comfortable are you with physical touch and closeness?
- What relationship patterns would you like to develop?

Daily Life:

- How does trauma impact your work or school performance?

- What activities or situations do you tend to avoid?
- How has your sense of safety in the world been affected?
- What aspects of daily life would you like to engage with more fully?

Resources and Strengths:

- What helps you feel calm and grounded?
- Who are your sources of support?
- What activities bring you joy or satisfaction?
- What personal strengths have helped you survive and cope?

Review your responses and notice patterns. This map isn't meant to catalogue everything wrong, but rather to provide a realistic assessment of where you are now and where you'd like to grow. Return to this worksheet periodically to track your progress.

The path of somatic healing requires patience, curiosity, and compassion for your own process. Your body has protected you through difficult experiences, and now it's ready to learn new ways of being in the world. The exercises and concepts in this chapter provide a foundation for the deeper work ahead. Trust your body's wisdom—it knows how to heal when given the right conditions and support.

Key Insights for Body Wisdom Development:

- Your body holds its own intelligence separate from your thinking mind
- Trauma creates protective patterns that once served you but may now limit you
- Healing happens through presence and awareness, not force or effort
- Each person's nervous system has its own timing and needs

- Small, consistent practices create more lasting change than dramatic interventions
- Your body's signals provide constant feedback about your internal state

Chapter 2: Building Your Foundation

Safety forms the bedrock of all somatic healing work. Without adequate safety—both internal and external—the nervous system remains locked in defensive patterns, making meaningful change impossible. This chapter addresses a fundamental truth that many therapeutic approaches overlook: you cannot heal from a place of threat or overwhelm. The nervous system must first recognize that survival is no longer at stake before it can access its natural capacity for restoration and growth.

Safety in somatic terms goes beyond physical protection. It encompasses the felt sense of being supported, the confidence that you can handle whatever arises in your internal experience, and the knowledge that you have choices about how to respond. Building this foundation requires patience and skill, but it makes all subsequent healing work possible.

Understanding Your Window of Tolerance

The window of tolerance, a concept developed by Dr. Dan Siegel, describes the zone of arousal where you can function optimally (8). Within this window, you can think clearly, respond flexibly to challenges, and maintain connection with others. When stress pushes you outside this window, you enter states of hyperarousal (fight/flight) or hypoarousal (freeze/collapse).

Everyone's window of tolerance varies in size and flexibility. Some people have naturally wide windows that allow them to handle significant stress while maintaining equilibrium. Others, particularly those with trauma histories, may have narrow windows that are easily exceeded by relatively minor stressors.

Consider the case of Michael, a 28-year-old paramedic whose window of tolerance had become extremely narrow following years of exposure to traumatic situations. What once felt manageable—traffic jams, work deadlines, family conflicts—now triggered intense reactions. He would either become explosively angry (hyperarousal) or shut down completely (hypoarousal), with very little middle ground.

Through somatic work, Michael learned to recognize the early signs of window violation. He noticed that his breathing became shallow and his shoulders tensed before he moved into hyperarousal. He also identified the foggy, disconnected feeling that preceded collapse into hypoarousal. Most importantly, he developed practices to support his nervous system before it became overwhelmed.

Michael's window gradually expanded as he practiced these regulation skills. He learned that expansion happened slowly and required consistent attention to his internal state. Some days his window felt wider; others, it contracted again. Rather than viewing this as failure, he learned to adjust his expectations and self-care practices based on his current capacity.

The edges of your window provide important information. When you notice yourself approaching hyperarousal, you can engage practices that support downregulation—slowing your breathing, feeling your feet on the ground, or engaging your parasympathetic nervous system through gentle movement. When you sense movement toward hypoarousal, you can use upregulating practices—opening your eyes wider, lengthening your spine, or engaging in mild physical activity.

Learning to track these states requires developing what somatic practitioners call "neuroception"—the ability to sense your nervous system state beneath the level of conscious thought. This skill improves with practice and becomes one of your most valuable tools for maintaining emotional equilibrium.

Creating Internal and External Safety

External safety involves creating environments and relationships that support your nervous system's natural capacity for regulation. This includes both physical safety—living in secure housing, having adequate resources, being free from violence or threat—and relational safety—having trustworthy people in your life who respond predictably and supportively.

However, many trauma survivors discover that even when external circumstances improve, they continue to feel unsafe internally. This occurs because trauma can dysregulate the nervous system's threat detection mechanisms, causing it to perceive danger even in neutral or safe situations.

Lisa, a survivor of domestic violence, found herself unable to relax even two years after leaving an abusive relationship. She lived in a safe apartment, had supportive friends, and worked in a peaceful environment, yet her nervous system remained hypervigilant. Loud sounds made her jump, unexpected phone calls triggered panic, and she found it difficult to sleep despite feeling exhausted.

Lisa's therapeutic work focused on helping her nervous system distinguish between past danger and present safety. She learned to orient to her current environment by consciously noticing details that confirmed her safety—the sound of children playing outside, the familiar smell of her coffee, the soft texture of her favorite blanket.

She also developed what somatic therapists call "resources"—internal and external supports that help regulate the nervous system. Her internal resources included memories of feeling loved and supported, images of peaceful places, and awareness of her own strength and resilience. External resources included her cat, certain pieces of music, and specific friends who made her feel calm and accepted.

Building internal safety often involves renegotiating your relationship with your own nervous system. Instead of viewing activation as something wrong that needs to be fixed, you learn to see it as information about your internal state. You develop curiosity about your responses rather than judgment, and you learn to support your system through difficult moments rather than fighting against them.

This process requires considerable self-compassion. Many trauma survivors have internalized messages that they should be "over it" by now or that their reactions are excessive. Learning to respond to yourself with kindness during moments of activation becomes a crucial aspect of building internal safety.

The Power of Co-regulation

Co-regulation describes the process by which nervous systems influence each other toward greater stability and calm. This occurs naturally in healthy relationships and forms the foundation for our ability to self-regulate later in life. Infants learn to manage their emotional states through co-regulation with caregivers; adults continue to benefit from co-regulating relationships throughout their lives (9).

For individuals with trauma histories, co-regulation can feel both deeply healing and intensely threatening. The very relationships that could provide nervous system support may trigger defensive responses based on past experiences of betrayal or harm.

David, a 45-year-old architect, grew up in a chaotic household where emotional regulation was impossible to predict. As an adult, he found himself simultaneously craving and avoiding close relationships. When someone offered comfort during distress, he often felt overwhelmed and needed to withdraw, even though part of him desperately wanted connection.

David's somatic work included learning to titrate co-regulation—experiencing small amounts of nervous system support from others without becoming overwhelmed. He started with very brief moments of connection—making eye contact with his therapist for just a few seconds, or sitting near a friend without conversation.

Gradually, David's tolerance for co-regulation increased. He learned to notice when his nervous system was ready for connection and when it needed space. He also developed the ability to communicate his needs to others, asking for specific types of support rather than hoping others would intuitively know what he needed.

Co-regulation can happen in many ways. Sometimes it involves direct interaction—synchronized breathing with another person, receiving appropriate touch, or simply being in the presence of someone who feels calm and grounded. Other times it occurs through connection with pets, nature, or even imagined relationships with supportive figures.

The key to beneficial co-regulation lies in choice and agency. When you feel forced to accept comfort or connection, your nervous system may respond defensively. When you can choose the timing, duration, and type of co-regulating experience, your system can more readily receive the support being offered.

When to Seek Professional Support

Somatic healing work can be profound and transformative, but it's not always appropriate to undertake alone. Certain signs indicate that professional support would be beneficial or necessary for safe progress.

Seek professional help if you experience:

- Dissociation that feels uncontrollable or interferes with daily functioning
- Thoughts of harming yourself or others
- Substance use that feels compulsive or out of control
- Flashbacks or intrusive memories that overwhelm your coping capacity
- Physical symptoms that haven't been medically evaluated
- Relationships that feel consistently unsafe or harmful

Also consider professional support if you find yourself repeatedly overwhelmed by the exercises in this workbook, or if exploring your trauma history triggers reactions that last for days or weeks. Healing trauma often requires the support of someone trained to recognize when you're approaching the edges of your capacity and who can help you slow down or modify your approach accordingly.

Professional somatic therapists receive extensive training in nervous system regulation, trauma physiology, and the subtleties of working with activation and shutdown. They can provide external regulation when your own system becomes overwhelmed, and they can guide you through territory that might be too challenging to navigate alone.

Finding a qualified somatic therapist requires some research. Look for practitioners who have completed training in established somatic modalities such as Somatic Experiencing, Hakomi, or Sensorimotor Psychotherapy. Many practitioners list their training on their websites or professional directories.

During initial consultations, pay attention to how your body responds to the therapist. Do you feel seen and understood? Does their presence feel calming or activating? Do they demonstrate understanding of trauma and nervous system functioning? Trust your somatic responses as much as your cognitive assessment of their qualifications.

Exercise 2.1: Establishing Your Safe Space Visualization

Creating a detailed internal safe space provides your nervous system with a resource you can access anytime you feel overwhelmed or dysregulated. This space can be real or imagined, indoors or outdoors, populated or solitary.

Settle into a comfortable position and close your eyes. Allow your breathing to find its natural rhythm. Begin to imagine a place where you feel completely safe and at peace. This might be a location from your past, somewhere you've visited, or a completely imagined environment.

Take time to develop rich sensory details about this space. What do you see around you? Notice colors, lighting, and visual textures. What sounds are present? Perhaps gentle wind, flowing water, or peaceful quiet. What do you smell? Fresh air, flowers, or the scent of your grandmother's kitchen?

How does your body feel in this space? Do you notice warmth from sunlight, coolness from shade, or the comfort of soft surfaces? What position is your body in? Are you sitting, lying down, standing, or moving?

Most importantly, what creates the sense of safety in this space? Is it the natural protection of mountains or trees? The presence of loving beings? The absence of threat? The feeling of being completely accepted and welcomed?

Spend 10-15 minutes exploring this safe space, allowing it to become as real and detailed as possible. Notice how your nervous system responds as you maintain connection with this image. You may feel your breathing deepen, your muscles relax, or a sense of calm settling through your body.

Before ending the visualization, establish a way to quickly return to this space when needed. This might involve focusing on one particular detail—the feeling of warm sand beneath your feet, the sound of gentle rain, or the image of protective mountains. Practice returning to this anchor several times.

You can revisit and modify this safe space anytime. Some people develop multiple safe spaces for different needs—one for energy and vitality, another for deep rest, another for creative inspiration. Trust your imagination and your nervous system's wisdom about what feels most supportive.

Exercise 2.2: Grounding Through the Five Senses

Grounding techniques help orient your nervous system to present-moment safety by engaging your senses with current, non-threatening stimuli. This exercise is particularly useful during moments of activation, dissociation, or overwhelm.

The 5-4-3-2-1 technique engages each sense systematically:

5 Things You Can See: Look around your environment and identify five specific visual details. Rather than just noticing "a tree," you might observe "the way sunlight creates patterns through the green leaves" or "the rough texture of brown bark." Spend 15-30 seconds with each visual detail, really allowing your eyes to explore.

4 Things You Can Touch: Identify four different textures or sensations you can feel. This might include the temperature of the air on your skin, the texture of your clothing, the firmness of your chair, or the smoothness of an object in your hands. Spend time really focusing on the tactile experience of each sensation.

3 Things You Can Hear: Listen for three distinct sounds in your environment. These might include traffic in the distance, birds singing, the hum of air conditioning, or the sound of your own breathing. Allow yourself to really focus on each sound without trying to block out others.

2 Things You Can Smell: Notice two different scents present in your environment. This might be coffee, fresh air, cleaning products, or your own perfume. If you can't detect distinct smells, you can create them by stepping outside, opening a window, or finding something with a pleasant scent.

1 Thing You Can Taste: Focus on one taste in your mouth. This might be lingering flavors from something you've consumed, or simply the neutral taste of your own mouth. You can also intentionally taste something—a mint, a sip of water, or a small piece of food.

Practice this technique when you feel calm so it becomes familiar and accessible during more challenging moments. You can also modify it by focusing more extensively on whichever sense feels most grounding to you, or by doing multiple rounds if needed.

Exercise 2.3: Building Your Resource Library

Resources are any experiences, memories, images, or practices that help your nervous system move toward regulation and calm. Building a diverse resource library provides you with multiple options for supporting yourself during difficult moments.

Create four categories of resources:

Sensory Resources: These engage your senses in ways that promote calm and safety. Examples include:

- Soft textures like a favorite blanket or pet's fur
- Calming scents like lavender or vanilla
- Soothing sounds like gentle music or nature recordings

- Comforting tastes like herbal tea or a favorite healthy snack
- Visual beauty like photos of loved ones or peaceful landscapes

Movement Resources: These involve physical activities that help regulate your nervous system:

- Gentle stretching or yoga poses
- Walking, especially in nature
- Dancing to favorite music
- Progressive muscle relaxation
- Simple exercises like shoulder rolls or neck stretches

Relational Resources: These involve connection with others, either in person or through memory:

- Phone calls with supportive friends or family
- Hugging a pet or loved one
- Looking at photos of people who care about you
- Remembering times when you felt loved and accepted
- Connecting with communities that share your values

Internal Resources: These are qualities, memories, or images that exist within you:

- Memories of times when you felt strong, capable, or proud
- Awareness of personal qualities like courage, kindness, or perseverance
- Images of places where you've felt peaceful and safe
- Spiritual or religious practices that provide comfort
- Mantras or phrases that remind you of your worth and strength

Spend time identifying specific resources in each category. Test them by bringing each resource to mind and noticing how your body responds. Effective resources typically create some sense of ease, expansion, or settling in your nervous system.

Write your resources down and keep the list accessible. Add new resources as you discover them, and notice which ones feel most helpful in different situations. Some resources work better for high activation; others are more effective for low energy or depression.

Worksheet: Safety Planning Template

Creating a comprehensive safety plan helps you prepare for challenging moments and ensures you have concrete steps to take when your nervous system becomes overwhelmed.

Warning Signs List the early indicators that your nervous system is becoming dysregulated:

Physical signs (tension, breathing changes, temperature shifts): Emotional signs (irritability, anxiety, numbness): Behavioral signs (isolation, reactivity, avoidance): Cognitive signs (racing thoughts, confusion, difficulty concentrating):

Immediate Safety Strategies Identify specific actions you can take when you notice warning signs:

Quick grounding techniques (3 specific methods): Breathing exercises you find helpful: Movement practices that calm your system: Sensory resources you can access immediately:

Environmental Modifications List ways you can modify your environment to support safety:

Changes to lighting, sound, or temperature: Items to have readily available: Spaces that feel most safe and supportive: People who provide co-regulating presence:

Professional Support Contacts Record important phone numbers and information:

Therapist or counselor: Crisis hotline numbers: Trusted friend or family member: Medical providers: Emergency contacts:

Extended Support Strategies Identify longer-term practices that build safety and resilience:

Daily practices that support regulation: Weekly activities that replenish your resources: Monthly or seasonal practices for deeper restoration: Professional services that support your ongoing healing:

Review and update this safety plan regularly. Share relevant portions with trusted friends, family members, or professionals who might support you during difficult times. Having a concrete plan reduces anxiety and provides your nervous system with the security of knowing you have specific resources available when needed.

Safety provides the foundation for all meaningful change. As you develop greater internal and external safety, your capacity for experiencing sensation, emotion, and aliveness naturally expands. The work of the following chapters builds upon this foundation, introducing practices that gradually increase your tolerance for activation while maintaining your connection to safety and choice.

Essential Safety Building Blocks:

- Your window of tolerance can expand with patient, consistent practice
- Internal safety develops through self-compassion and nervous system awareness
- Co-regulation with others supports your individual healing capacity

- Professional support provides additional safety during challenging terrain
- Resources and safety plans create structure for navigating difficult moments
- Safety is not a destination but an ongoing practice of self-attunement

Chapter 3: Developing Body Literacy

Your body speaks in a language far more ancient and immediate than words—the language of sensation. Every moment of every day, your nervous system generates a constant stream of information about your internal state, your relationship to the environment, and your readiness for various activities. Learning to understand this somatic vocabulary transforms how you navigate emotional challenges, make decisions, and care for yourself.

Most people have some awareness of obvious sensations—hunger, fatigue, pain, or temperature. However, the subtle communications of the nervous system often go unnoticed or misinterpreted. The tightness in your chest before a difficult conversation, the settling in your belly when you're with someone trustworthy, the restless energy that signals readiness for change—these quiet messages contain guidance that no external advisor could provide.

Developing body literacy requires patience and practice. In a culture that prioritizes thinking over feeling, many people have learned to override or ignore their somatic experience. Reconnecting with this internal wisdom takes time, but it provides access to information that makes life more satisfying, relationships more authentic, and decisions more aligned with your true needs.

Sensation vs. Emotion vs. Thought

The distinction between sensation, emotion, and thought often seems artificial, since these experiences typically occur simultaneously and influence each other continuously. However, learning to differentiate between them provides valuable precision in understanding your internal experience and responding appropriately to different types of information.

Sensations are the raw data of physical experience—pressure, temperature, movement, texture, vibration, or spatial awareness. They occur in the body and can be located specifically: "I feel tightness in my throat," or "There's a fluttering sensation in my stomach." Sensations change constantly and provide immediate feedback about your current state.

Emotions emerge from the meaning your nervous system assigns to sensations within a particular context (10). Fear might manifest as rapid heartbeat, shallow breathing, and muscle tension, but these same sensations could be interpreted as excitement in a different context. Emotions typically have recognizable names—joy, anger, sadness, fear—and often carry impulses toward specific actions.

Thoughts are the cognitive interpretations, stories, and meanings you create about sensations and emotions. They often take the form of words or images and can either support or conflict with your somatic experience. For example, you might think "I should be happy about this promotion" while your body signals anxiety about increased responsibility.

Consider the case of Rebecca, a 29-year-old social worker who struggled with what she called "irrational anxiety." She would suddenly feel overwhelmed in social situations that seemed perfectly normal and safe. Through somatic work, Rebecca learned to distinguish between different layers of her experience.

She began noticing that her "anxiety" actually started with specific sensations—a slight tightening around her eyes, a quickening of her breath, and a subtle urge to scan the room for exits. These sensations occurred before she felt anxious emotionally or thought anxious thoughts.

As Rebecca developed more precision in tracking these sensations, she discovered they often signaled legitimate concerns about social dynamics that her conscious mind hadn't yet recognized. The eye tension occurred when someone in the group felt emotionally unsafe to her. The breathing changes happened when conversations became competitive or aggressive. The scanning behavior emerged when she sensed manipulation or dishonesty.

Rather than "irrational anxiety," Rebecca was experiencing her nervous system's sophisticated social radar. By learning to trust and interpret these somatic signals, she became much more skilled at navigating social situations and protecting her emotional well-being.

This level of discernment requires practice. Many people initially experience their internal world as an undifferentiated soup of sensation, emotion, and thought. Learning to separate these streams of information takes time but provides increasingly precise guidance for decision-making and self-care.

The SIBAM Model

SIBAM—Sensation, Image, Behavior, Affect, and Meaning—provides a framework for understanding how traumatic experiences become organized in the nervous system and how healing occurs through reorganizing these elements (11). Originally developed by Pat Ogden and her colleagues, this model helps track the different channels through which experience flows and provides multiple entry points for therapeutic intervention.

Sensation includes all physical experiences—heart rate, muscle tension, temperature, pressure, vibration, and spatial awareness. In trauma, certain sensations may become associated with danger and trigger defensive responses even in safe contexts.

Image encompasses visual, auditory, olfactory, gustatory, and kinesthetic memories or fantasies. Trauma survivors often experience intrusive images related to their experiences, but positive images can also serve as powerful resources for healing.

Behavior includes both external actions—posture, movement, gestures, facial expressions—and internal impulses toward action. Trauma can create both compulsive behaviors and protective inhibitions that once served survival but may now limit functioning.

Affect refers to emotional states and feelings. Trauma often creates emotional dysregulation, with feelings becoming either overwhelming floods or numbed absence. Healing involves developing capacity to experience a full range of emotions without becoming overwhelmed.

Meaning includes thoughts, beliefs, interpretations, and stories about experience. Trauma can create limiting beliefs about self, others, and the world that persist long after the original threat has passed.

Consider the case of Tony, a 38-year-old construction worker who developed panic attacks after falling from scaffolding. Though he wasn't seriously injured, his nervous system remained activated by heights and confined spaces.

Using the SIBAM model, Tony and his therapist mapped his panic responses:

Sensation: Racing heart, sweating, muscle tension, dizziness
Image: Visual memory of looking down from the scaffolding, imagined scenarios of falling **Behavior:** Avoiding heights, gripping railings tightly, scanning for escape routes **Affect:** Fear, helplessness, anger at himself for being "weak" **Meaning:** "I'm not safe," "I can't trust my body," "I'm not the capable person I used to be"

Rather than trying to eliminate these responses, Tony learned to work with each channel of experience. He practiced grounding techniques to shift his sensations from panic to stability. He developed positive images of successfully completing projects and being supported by coworkers. He learned behavioral techniques for gradually re-engaging with heights while maintaining choice and control.

Tony also explored the emotions beneath his panic—grief for his lost sense of invincibility, anger about the dangerous working conditions, and fear about his family's financial security. As he processed these feelings, his panic responses naturally decreased.

Finally, Tony examined the meanings he had created about the accident. He realized he had developed beliefs about personal failure that weren't supported by evidence. The scaffolding had been improperly secured by someone else; his fall was not due to incompetence or carelessness. Recognizing this helped him reclaim his sense of professional competence.

The SIBAM model demonstrates that healing can begin through any channel of experience. Sometimes working with sensation provides the most direct route to change. Other times, shifting behavior or meaning creates the opening for nervous system reorganization. Effective somatic therapy moves fluidly between these different channels, following the client's natural healing process.

Tracking Activation and Deactivation

Your nervous system constantly moves between states of activation and deactivation, responding to internal and external cues about safety and threat. Learning to track these movements provides valuable information about your current capacity and helps you make choices that support optimal functioning.

Activation occurs when your nervous system perceives challenge or threat and mobilizes energy for response. Healthy activation feels energizing and purposeful—the alert focus before an important presentation, the physical readiness for athletic performance, or the excitement of creative inspiration. Problematic activation feels overwhelming, chaotic, or disconnected from current circumstances.

Deactivation involves the nervous system's movement toward rest, restoration, and integration. Healthy deactivation feels peaceful and restorative—the deep relaxation after completing a project, the quiet contentment of spending time in nature, or the settling that occurs during meditation. Problematic deactivation feels like collapse, numbness, or disconnection from life energy.

The key to nervous system health lies not in remaining constantly calm, but in developing flexibility to move appropriately between activation and deactivation based on current needs and circumstances.

Elena, a 42-year-old nurse, came to therapy exhausted from years of working in a high-stress hospital environment. She described feeling either "completely wired" or "totally wiped out," with little middle ground between these states.

Elena learned to track the early signs of healthy activation—increased alertness, purposeful energy, clear thinking—versus unhealthy hyperactivation—racing thoughts, muscle tension, irritability. She also distinguished between restorative deactivation—relaxed breathing, soft muscles, present-moment awareness—and problematic hypoactivation—flatness, disconnection, or inability to engage with life.

By monitoring these states throughout her workday, Elena discovered patterns she hadn't previously noticed. Her hyperactivation often began during specific types of medical emergencies that reminded her of her father's death in a hospital.

Her hypoactivation typically followed interactions with particular colleagues who reminded her of her critical mother.

This awareness allowed Elena to develop targeted interventions. When she noticed early signs of hyperactivation, she could take brief breaks to ground herself, adjust her breathing, or request support from teammates. When she sensed movement toward hypoactivation, she could engage in mild physical activity, connect with colleagues she enjoyed, or remind herself of meaningful aspects of her work.

Elena also learned to honor her nervous system's natural rhythms rather than fighting against them. Some days she had more capacity for activation; others required more rest and restoration. By working with these patterns rather than forcing herself into a consistent state, she found her overall energy and job satisfaction improved significantly.

Understanding Your Nervous System States

The autonomic nervous system operates through three main branches that govern different aspects of physiological and psychological functioning (12). Understanding these states helps you recognize your current capacity and choose appropriate responses to life circumstances.

Sympathetic Activation mobilizes energy for action through the fight-or-flight response. When functioning optimally, this system provides energy for meeting challenges, engaging in physical activity, and responding to genuine threats. Signs of healthy sympathetic activation include:

- Increased heart rate and breathing
- Enhanced alertness and focus
- Mobilized energy and readiness for action
- Clear thinking and good coordination

When dysregulated, sympathetic activation becomes hyperactivation, characterized by:

- Racing heart and shallow breathing
- Anxiety, panic, or rage
- Scattered thinking and poor coordination
- Feeling overwhelmed or out of control

Parasympathetic Activation supports rest, restoration, and social connection. The ventral vagal branch of this system promotes states of calm alertness, creativity, and social engagement. Signs of healthy parasympathetic activation include:

- Calm, deep breathing
- Relaxed muscle tone
- Present-moment awareness
- Openness to connection with others

Dorsal Vagal Activation is an older parasympathetic system that promotes shutdown and conservation of energy when threats feel insurmountable. In small doses, this system supports deep rest and restoration. When chronic or extreme, it creates:

- Numbness and disconnection
- Low energy and motivation
- Difficulty thinking clearly
- Sense of hopelessness or despair

Marcus, a 35-year-old teacher, struggled with what he called "emotional whiplash"—rapidly cycling between states of high stress and complete shutdown. Some days he felt energized and capable; others, he could barely get out of bed.

Through somatic work, Marcus learned to recognize these as different nervous system states rather than character flaws or mood disorders. His hyperactivation typically occurred in response to work stress, family conflicts, or financial worries. His shutdown often followed periods of sustained hyperactivation, particularly when he felt unable to address the underlying stressors.

Marcus developed practices for each state. When hyperactivated, he used breathing exercises, gentle movement, and conscious muscle relaxation to support his nervous system's return to calm alertness. When in shutdown, he practiced very gentle activation through mild exercise, social connection, or engaging in activities that brought him small amounts of pleasure.

Most importantly, Marcus learned to recognize his optimal state—calm but alert, energized but not overwhelmed, present but not hypervigilant. He noticed that this state occurred most easily when he felt a sense of choice and control over his circumstances, when he had adequate rest and nutrition, and when he maintained connection with supportive people.

By tracking these patterns, Marcus could make environmental and lifestyle adjustments that supported his nervous system's natural capacity for regulation. His emotional volatility decreased significantly as he learned to work with his autonomic responses rather than fighting against them.

Exercise 3.1: Sensation Vocabulary Building

Developing precise language for physical sensations enhances your ability to track and communicate about your internal experience. This exercise expands your somatic vocabulary through systematic exploration.

Settle into a comfortable position and close your eyes. Begin with several deep breaths, allowing your attention to settle into your body. For this exercise, you'll systematically explore different qualities of sensation.

Temperature Sensations: Bring your attention to different areas of your body and notice temperature variations. You might find:

- Warmth or heat
- Coolness or cold
- Areas that feel neutral
- Places where temperature seems to shift or move

Spend 2-3 minutes exploring temperature, noticing both obvious and subtle variations.

Pressure and Density Sensations: Now focus on experiences of pressure, weight, or density:

- Heaviness or lightness
- Pressure or spaciousness
- Density or emptiness
- Compression or expansion

Notice how these qualities may differ in various parts of your body.

Movement and Energy Sensations: Observe any sense of movement, flow, or energy:

- Flowing or stuck
- Moving or still
- Vibrating or calm
- Pulsing or steady
- Rising or sinking

Texture and Quality Sensations: Explore more subtle qualitative aspects:

- Smooth or rough
- Soft or hard

- Sharp or dull
- Tight or loose
- Tingling or numb

Size and Shape Sensations: Notice spatial qualities of different body areas:

- Large or small
- Expanded or contracted
- Round or angular
- Open or closed

After exploring each category, take a few minutes to sense your body as a whole. Notice which sensations drew your attention most strongly and which were more difficult to detect.

Keep a sensation journal for one week, noting different physical experiences throughout each day. Use the vocabulary from this exercise to describe your observations with increasing precision. You may notice that certain sensations correlate with particular emotions, thoughts, or life circumstances.

Exercise 3.2: Daily Sensation Tracking Practice

Consistent tracking builds your capacity to notice subtle changes in your internal state and respond appropriately to your body's communications. This practice involves brief, regular check-ins with your somatic experience.

Set reminders on your phone for four times throughout the day—morning, midday, late afternoon, and evening. When the reminder sounds, pause whatever you're doing for 60-90 seconds and complete this quick assessment.

General Body Awareness: Take three conscious breaths and ask yourself:

- How does my body feel right now overall?
- What draws my attention first?
- What's the general quality of energy or aliveness in my system?

Specific Region Check: Quickly scan these areas, noting the first sensation you notice in each:

- Head and face
- Neck and shoulders
- Chest and upper back
- Arms and hands
- Abdomen
- Lower back and hips
- Legs and feet

Nervous System State: Assess your current autonomic state:

- Do I feel calm, activated, or shut down?
- Is my energy moving toward activity or rest?
- How available am I for connection with others?
- What does my body need right now?

Environmental Response: Notice how your body is responding to your current environment:

- Does this space feel supportive or stressful?
- How is my body positioned? Does this position feel good?
- What environmental factors (light, sound, temperature, people) affect my comfort?

Record your observations in a simple log. After one week, review your entries for patterns. You might notice:

- Certain times of day when you feel most or least comfortable

- Environmental factors that consistently affect your well-being
- Early warning signs of stress or overwhelm
- Activities or situations that support your nervous system regulation

This information helps you make informed decisions about self-care, scheduling, and environmental modifications that support your optimal functioning.

Exercise 3.3: Pendulation - Riding the Waves

Pendulation describes the natural movement of the nervous system between activation and deactivation, expansion and contraction, pleasure and discomfort. Learning to support this natural rhythm enhances your capacity to experience intensity without becoming overwhelmed.

Begin in a comfortable seated position with your eyes closed. Take several minutes to settle into your body using the body scan technique from previous exercises.

Identify Contrasting Sensations: Notice two different areas of your body that feel distinctly different from each other. For example:

- One area that feels tense and another that feels relaxed
- One area that feels warm and another that feels cool
- One area that feels heavy and another that feels light
- One area that feels uncomfortable and another that feels pleasant

Focus on the More Challenging Sensation: Bring your attention to whichever sensation feels more intense, uncomfortable, or activating. Notice exactly what you experience there without trying to change it. Observe:

- The precise quality of the sensation
- Whether it stays the same or shifts as you observe it
- Any impulses to move away from or change the sensation

Stay with this sensation for 30-60 seconds, or until you notice any natural shift or change.

Shift to the More Comfortable Sensation: Now move your attention to the area that feels more pleasant, relaxed, or neutral. Allow yourself to fully receive whatever comfort or ease is available there. Notice:

- How your nervous system responds to this more pleasant experience
- Whether the sensation deepens or expands as you focus on it
- Any sense of relief, settling, or integration

Remain with this sensation for 30-60 seconds.

Continue Pendulating: Slowly move your attention back and forth between these two areas, spending 30-60 seconds with each. Notice:

- How the sensations may change as you pendulate between them
- Whether the contrast between them becomes more or less pronounced
- Any overall shifts in your nervous system state

Complete Integration: End by sensing both areas simultaneously, or by allowing your attention to include your whole body. Notice any changes from when you began the exercise.

Practice pendulation regularly with different sensation pairs. This technique helps build tolerance for intensity while maintaining connection to resources and supports the nervous system's natural capacity for self-regulation.

Exercise 3.4: Noticing Without Changing

One of the most challenging yet essential skills in somatic work involves observing your internal experience without immediately trying to fix, change, or improve it. This practice builds capacity for being present with difficulty and supports the nervous system's natural healing processes.

Find a quiet place where you won't be disturbed for 15-20 minutes. Sit comfortably with your eyes closed and spend a few minutes settling into your body.

Choose a Mild Challenge: Select something in your current experience that feels slightly uncomfortable or challenging, but not overwhelming. This might be:

- A physical sensation like tension, restlessness, or fatigue
- An emotional state like anxiety, sadness, or irritation
- A mental state like worry, confusion, or boredom

Begin with Curious Observation: Bring your attention to this experience with an attitude of gentle curiosity rather than judgment or problem-solving. Ask yourself:

- What exactly am I experiencing right now?
- Where do I feel this in my body?
- What are the specific qualities of this sensation or state?

Notice the Impulse to Change: Observe any urges that arise to:

- Fix or eliminate the uncomfortable experience
- Distract yourself or move away from it

- Judge yourself for having this experience
- Figure out why it's happening or what it means

Simply notice these impulses without acting on them.

Practice Pure Witnessing: For several minutes, practice simply being present with the challenging experience without trying to modify it in any way. If you notice yourself slipping into problem-solving mode, gently return to pure observation.

Notice:

- Does the sensation stay exactly the same, or does it shift naturally?
- What happens when you stop trying to change your experience?
- Can you find any interest or curiosity about this internal state?

Track Any Natural Changes: Often, when we stop trying to force change, transformation occurs spontaneously. Notice:

- Any shifts in intensity, location, or quality of the sensation
- Changes in your emotional relationship to the experience
- Moments of natural settling, shifting, or integration

End with Appreciation: Complete the exercise by appreciating your willingness to be present with difficulty. This capacity for presence is one of the most healing gifts you can offer yourself.

Start with very mild challenges and gradually work with more intense experiences as your capacity develops. This practice builds the foundation for all other somatic work.

Worksheet: Personal Sensation Dictionary

Creating your personal sensation dictionary helps you develop precision in tracking and communicating about your internal experience. Complete this worksheet over several days or weeks, adding entries as you notice new sensations.

Pleasant Sensations: List physical sensations that feel good, comfortable, or supportive:

Location: _____ Description: _____
When it occurs: _____ What supports it: _____

(Create multiple entries for different pleasant sensations)

Neutral Sensations: Record sensations that feel neither pleasant nor unpleasant:

Location: _____ Description: _____
When it occurs: _____ Context: _____

Challenging Sensations: Identify difficult sensations without judgment:

Location: _____ Description: _____
Triggers or context: _____ What helps: _____

Movement and Energy Sensations: Track sensations related to energy, movement, or aliveness:

Type of movement/energy: _____ Location: _____ Quality (fast/slow, smooth/jerky, etc.): _____ When it occurs: _____

Warning Signal Sensations: List sensations that serve as early warning signs of stress or overwhelm:

Sensation: _____ Location: _____
What it signals: _____ What helps when you notice it: _____

Resource Sensations: Identify sensations that indicate safety, calm, or well-being:

Sensation: _____ Location: _____ How to cultivate it: _____ When you feel it most: _____

_____

Relationship Between Sensations and Emotions: Note connections you observe between physical sensations and emotional states:

Emotion: _____ Associated sensation: _____ Location: _____ Pattern or timing: _____

Review your dictionary regularly and continue adding entries. This document becomes a valuable reference for understanding your unique somatic patterns and developing personalized regulation strategies.

Building Your Somatic Foundation

Developing body literacy creates the foundation for all subsequent healing work. As you become more skilled at tracking sensation, distinguishing between different types of internal experience, and supporting your nervous system's natural rhythms, you develop a reliable internal guidance system that can inform decisions large and small.

This foundation of somatic awareness prepares you for the more active practices in the following chapters. With your growing ability to track and tolerate sensation, you're ready to explore how conscious breathing, movement, touch, and sound can support your nervous system's capacity for regulation and resilience.

Core Elements of Body Literacy:

- Sensations provide constant information about your internal state and needs
- Learning to distinguish between sensation, emotion, and thought creates precision
- The SIBAM model offers multiple pathways for understanding and healing trauma
- Tracking activation and deactivation patterns reveals your optimal functioning zones
- Understanding nervous system states helps you respond appropriately to your capacity
- Practicing presence without changing builds tolerance for life's challenges
- Your personal sensation vocabulary becomes a guide for self-care and decision-making

Chapter 4: Conscious Breathing for Healing

Your breath holds extraordinary power to transform your nervous system in real time. Unlike other bodily functions that operate automatically—your heartbeat, digestion, or temperature regulation—breathing exists in a unique space between voluntary and involuntary control. You can consciously direct your breath, yet it continues without your attention. This dual nature makes breathing an ideal gateway for healing trauma and building nervous system resilience.

Each breath creates a direct pathway to influence your autonomic nervous system. Through specific breathing patterns, you can activate your parasympathetic nervous system to promote calm, engage your sympathetic system for healthy energy, or help discharge trapped activation from traumatic experiences. The beauty of breathwork lies in its accessibility—you always have your breath available as a tool for regulation and healing.

The Science of Breathwork and Trauma

Trauma fundamentally alters breathing patterns. When faced with threat, the nervous system prioritizes survival over optimal breathing, leading to shallow, restricted, or irregular patterns that can persist long after danger has passed (13). These altered patterns maintain the body in a state of chronic stress, limiting access to calm, clear thinking, and emotional regulation.

Research demonstrates that conscious breathing practices directly affect brain chemistry and nervous system function. Slow, rhythmic breathing stimulates the vagus nerve, increasing production of GABA (gamma-aminobutyric acid), the brain's primary calming neurotransmitter (14). This same breathing pattern activates the parasympathetic nervous system, promoting rest, digestion, and healing.

Dr. Elissa Epel's research at UCSF shows that controlled breathing practices can reduce cortisol levels, improve heart rate variability, and increase telomerase activity—an enzyme associated with cellular longevity and stress resistance (15). These changes occur within minutes of beginning conscious breathing practices, making breathwork one of the most immediate interventions available for nervous system regulation.

Consider the case of Jennifer, a 31-year-old paramedic who developed panic attacks after responding to a series of traumatic emergency calls. Her breathing had become chronically shallow and rapid, keeping her nervous system locked in hyperarousal. Even during calm moments, she felt anxious and on edge.

Jennifer's therapist taught her to track her breathing patterns throughout the day. She discovered that her breath remained consistently shallow and confined to her upper chest. During panic attacks, her breathing became even more restricted, creating a cycle where poor breathing increased anxiety, which further compromised her breathing.

Through systematic breathwork training, Jennifer learned to expand her breathing capacity gradually. She started with simple awareness exercises, then progressed to techniques that engaged her diaphragm and expanded her ribcage. As her breathing patterns normalized, her panic attacks decreased in both frequency and intensity.

The transformation took several months of consistent practice. Jennifer noticed that when she maintained conscious breathing during work shifts, she felt more centered and less reactive to stressful situations. Her colleagues remarked that she seemed calmer and more present. Most importantly, Jennifer regained confidence in her ability to regulate her own nervous system.

Different Breathing Patterns and Their Effects

Your breathing pattern directly communicates with your nervous system, signaling safety or threat based on the rhythm, depth, and location of each breath. Understanding these signals allows you to consciously choose breathing patterns that support your desired state of mind and body.

Shallow, rapid breathing (more than 16 breaths per minute) signals threat to your nervous system, activating sympathetic responses even in safe environments. This pattern occurs naturally during genuine emergencies but becomes problematic when it persists chronically. Many trauma survivors develop this pattern as a protective mechanism that no longer serves them.

Slow, deep breathing (6-8 breaths per minute) activates parasympathetic responses, promoting calm, clear thinking, and emotional regulation. This pattern enhances heart rate variability, improves oxygen delivery to tissues, and supports optimal brain function. Most people find this breathing rate naturally relaxing and restorative.

Coherent breathing (5 breaths per minute) creates optimal heart rate variability and nervous system balance. This specific rhythm synchronizes heart rate, blood pressure, and brain wave patterns, creating a state of physiological coherence that supports both calm alertness and emotional resilience.

Extended exhale breathing (exhale longer than inhale) specifically activates the parasympathetic nervous system through stimulation of the vagus nerve. This pattern is particularly effective for reducing anxiety, promoting sleep, and calming hyperarousal states.

Energizing breathing (inhale longer than exhale or rapid, controlled breathing) can safely activate the sympathetic nervous system when more energy or alertness is needed. These patterns are useful for combating depression, increasing motivation, or preparing for challenging activities.

Carlos, a 44-year-old accountant, experienced chronic fatigue and depression following a difficult divorce. His breathing had become consistently slow and shallow, reflecting his hypoaroused nervous system state. He felt exhausted despite adequate sleep and struggled to find motivation for daily activities.

Carlos learned to use activating breathing patterns to energize his system when needed. He practiced techniques that emphasized longer inhalations and shorter exhalations, gradually building his capacity for healthy activation. He also used rapid, controlled breathing exercises to generate energy for exercise and social activities.

The key for Carlos was learning to match his breathing practice to his current needs rather than using the same technique regardless of his state. On days when he felt anxious or overwhelmed, he used calming breath patterns. When he felt flat or disconnected, he chose energizing techniques. This flexibility allowed him to support his nervous system's movement toward balance.

Within three months of consistent practice, Carlos noticed significant improvements in his energy levels and mood. He still experienced some days of low energy, but these became less frequent and less severe. His breathing had become a reliable tool for influencing his emotional and physical state.

Breath as a Bridge Between Voluntary and Involuntary

Breathing occupies a unique position in human physiology as the only autonomic function that can be consciously controlled. This characteristic makes it an ideal bridge between conscious intention and unconscious healing processes. Through breath, you can access and influence parts of your nervous system that typically operate outside of conscious awareness.

The diaphragm, your primary breathing muscle, connects to the vagus nerve—the longest cranial nerve that influences heart rate, digestion, immune function, and emotional regulation. When you breathe deeply and engage your diaphragm fully, you directly stimulate this nerve, promoting parasympathetic activation and healing responses throughout your body.

Your breathing pattern also affects brainwave states. Slow, rhythmic breathing promotes alpha waves associated with relaxed alertness and creativity. Rapid breathing can induce beta waves linked to focused attention, while extremely slow breathing may generate theta waves connected to deep relaxation and integration.

Patricia, a 52-year-old teacher, struggled with insomnia following the death of her mother. Her grief felt overwhelming, and she found herself unable to relax even when exhausted. Her mind raced with memories and worries, preventing restful sleep.

Patricia learned to use her breath as a bridge to influence her unconscious processes. She practiced breathing techniques specifically designed to promote sleep—patterns that slowed her heart rate, activated her parasympathetic nervous system, and shifted her brainwave state toward relaxation.

Initially, Patricia found it difficult to maintain focus on her breathing. Her mind kept returning to her grief and worries. Her therapist taught her to use these distractions as part of the practice rather than obstacles to overcome. Each time her mind wandered, she gently returned attention to her breath, gradually building her capacity for sustained attention.

Over time, Patricia's nervous system learned to associate specific breathing patterns with sleep preparation. She developed a bedtime routine that included breathwork, and her sleep quality gradually improved. The breathing practice didn't eliminate her grief, but it gave her nervous system the support it needed to process her loss while maintaining basic functioning.

Exercise 4.1: Three-Dimensional Breathing

This foundational exercise builds full breathing capacity by engaging all areas of your lungs and ribcage. Many people breathe primarily with their upper chest, limiting oxygen intake and maintaining sympathetic nervous system activation. Three-dimensional breathing restores natural, full breathing patterns.

Sit comfortably with your back straight but not rigid. Place one hand on your chest and one hand on your belly. Close your eyes and observe your natural breathing pattern for several breaths without trying to change it.

Phase 1: Belly Breathing Begin by breathing into your lower abdomen, allowing your belly to expand on the inhale and contract on the exhale. The hand on your chest should remain relatively still while the hand on your belly moves. Practice this for 5-10 breaths, focusing on expanding your abdomen in all directions—forward, to the sides, and toward your back.

Phase 2: Rib Breathing Place your hands on the sides of your ribcage. Breathe into this middle area of your torso, feeling your ribs expand outward like an accordion. Your belly and chest should remain relatively quiet while your middle ribs move outward on the inhale and inward on the exhale. Practice for 5-10 breaths.

Phase 3: Chest Breathing Return one hand to your upper chest. Breathe into this area, feeling your upper ribs and collarbone gently rise on the inhale and settle on the exhale. Keep this movement subtle—avoid forcing or exaggerating the chest expansion. Practice for 5-10 breaths.

Phase 4: Three-Dimensional Integration Now combine all three areas into one smooth, continuous breath. Inhale by expanding first your belly, then your ribs, then your chest. Exhale by gently releasing first your chest, then your ribs, then your belly. The entire movement should feel like a wave flowing through your torso.

Practice this integrated breathing for 10-15 breaths. If you feel lightheaded, return to normal breathing for a few breaths before continuing. End by observing your natural breathing pattern and noticing any changes from when you began.

Practice three-dimensional breathing daily, ideally at the same time each day. Most people find it easiest to establish this practice upon waking or before sleep. Start with 5-10 minutes and gradually increase the duration as your capacity develops.

Exercise 4.2: Coherent Breathing (5-5 Rhythm)

Coherent breathing creates optimal heart rate variability and nervous system balance through a specific rhythm of 5 seconds inhale and 5 seconds exhale. This pattern produces approximately 6 breaths per minute, which research shows generates maximum coherence between heart rate, blood pressure, and nervous system function.

Find a comfortable position where you can breathe freely. You can practice sitting, lying down, or even walking slowly. Close your eyes or soften your gaze downward.

Establishing the Rhythm Begin by breathing naturally for several breaths. Then slowly extend your inhale to a count of 5 and your exhale to a count of 5. Count at whatever pace feels comfortable—the goal is equal timing, not a specific speed.

If 5 seconds feels too long initially, start with 4-4 or even 3-3 and gradually build up to 5-5. If 5 seconds feels easy, you can experiment with 6-6 or 7-7, but most people find 5-5 optimal for coherence.

Maintaining Natural Ease The breathing should feel smooth and effortless rather than forced or strained. You're not trying to take the deepest possible breaths, but rather to establish a comfortable, sustainable rhythm. The breath should feel natural within this timing structure.

Focus on making the transitions between inhale and exhale smooth rather than abrupt. Avoid holding your breath between phases—let the inhale flow naturally into the exhale and vice versa.

Adding Heart Focus (Optional) If you feel comfortable with the basic rhythm, you can add attention to your heart area. Place your hand on your chest and imagine breathing directly into and out of your heart. This heart focus can enhance the coherence effects of the breathing pattern.

Some people find it helpful to imagine breathing in positive qualities like peace or gratitude and breathing out stress or tension. Others prefer to maintain simple attention to the breath rhythm without adding mental content.

Duration and Integration Practice coherent breathing for 5-20 minutes, depending on your experience and available time. Even 3-5 minutes can produce beneficial effects. You may notice increased calm, mental clarity, or physical relaxation during or after the practice.

End by returning to natural breathing and sitting quietly for a minute or two. Notice any changes in your physical sensations, emotional state, or mental clarity.

This technique can be practiced anytime you want to promote nervous system balance—before important meetings, during stressful situations, or as part of your daily self-care routine.

Exercise 4.3: The Physiological Sigh

The physiological sigh is a natural breathing pattern that your nervous system uses to downregulate stress and promote calm. Dr. Andrew Huberman's research at Stanford demonstrates that this specific pattern—a double inhale followed by a long exhale—is the fastest way to calm your nervous system in real time (16).

This breathing pattern occurs naturally when you're transitioning from stress to relaxation—you might notice it spontaneously after completing a challenging task or during moments of relief. By practicing it consciously, you can trigger this calming response whenever needed.

The Basic Pattern Sit or stand comfortably with your spine straight. Take a normal inhale through your nose, then take a second, smaller inhale on top of the first one—like you're sipping a bit more air. This double inhale fully inflates all the air sacs in your lungs.

Follow this with a long, slow exhale through your mouth, making the exhale much longer than the combined inhales. The exhale should feel like a gentle sigh or like you're slowly deflating a balloon.

Timing and Rhythm The first inhale might take 2-3 seconds, the second small inhale adds another 1-2 seconds, and the exhale should last 6-8 seconds or longer. The exact timing is less important than the pattern—double inhale through the nose, long exhale through the mouth.

Focus on making the exhale as long and complete as feels comfortable. This extended exhale activates your parasympathetic nervous system and stimulates the vagus nerve, promoting immediate relaxation.

When to Use This Technique The physiological sigh is particularly effective for:

- Acute stress or anxiety
- Moments of frustration or anger
- After difficult conversations or situations
- When feeling overwhelmed or panicked
- Before sleep to promote relaxation
- During any transition from high stress to calm

Practice Guidelines You can repeat the physiological sigh 1-3 times in sequence, then return to normal breathing. Most people notice immediate effects after just one cycle, but you can repeat it as needed.

This technique is safe for almost everyone and can be used multiple times throughout the day. It's particularly useful because it works quickly and can be done discreetly in most situations.

Unlike longer breathing practices, the physiological sigh is designed for immediate relief rather than extended practice. Use it as a tool for acute stress management rather than a daily meditation practice.

Exercise 4.4: Breath for Activation and Calming

Learning to use specific breathing patterns to either energize or calm your nervous system gives you precise tools for state regulation. This exercise teaches two contrasting techniques that you can choose based on your current needs and desired outcome.

Calming Breath Pattern (Extended Exhale) This pattern activates your parasympathetic nervous system and promotes relaxation by making your exhale longer than your inhale.

Sit comfortably and breathe naturally for several breaths. Then begin breathing with this pattern: inhale for 4 counts, exhale for 6 counts. If this feels comfortable, you can extend to inhale for 4 counts, exhale for 8 counts.

Focus on making the exhale slow and controlled rather than forced. You can exhale through your nose or mouth—experiment to see which feels more calming for you. Some people find that pursing their lips slightly during the exhale creates a more controlled and calming breath.

Practice this pattern for 10-20 breaths or until you notice a shift toward greater calm. This technique is particularly effective for anxiety, insomnia, or when you need to transition from activity to rest.

Energizing Breath Pattern (Extended Inhale) This pattern gently activates your sympathetic nervous system and can increase energy and alertness by emphasizing the inhale.

Start with natural breathing, then shift to this pattern: inhale for 6 counts, exhale for 4 counts. You can also try inhale for 8 counts, exhale for 4 counts if the first ratio feels too easy.

Make the inhale full and expansive, feeling your ribcage widen and your lungs fill completely. The exhale should be complete but not forced or extended. Focus on the expansion and fullness of each inhale.

Practice for 10-20 breaths or until you notice increased alertness or energy. This technique is useful for depression, fatigue, or when you need to increase motivation and focus.

Choosing the Right Pattern Learn to assess your current state before choosing which breathing pattern to use. If you feel anxious, overwhelmed, or hyperactivated, use the calming pattern. If you feel tired, depressed, or unmotivated, try the energizing pattern.

You can also use these patterns strategically—energizing breath in the morning to start your day or before exercise, calming breath in the evening to prepare for sleep or after stressful situations.

Exercise 4.5: Voo Breath for Vagus Nerve

The Voo breath, developed by Dr. Peter Levine, specifically stimulates the vagus nerve and promotes nervous system regulation through vocal vibration. The sound "Voo" creates vibrations in your chest that massage the vagus nerve, promoting parasympathetic activation and discharge of trapped stress energy.

This exercise combines conscious breathing with vocal expression, making it particularly effective for releasing stress and trauma that may be stored in your nervous system. The vibration helps complete stress responses that may have been interrupted during traumatic experiences.

Basic Voo Breath Technique Sit comfortably with your spine straight or lie down if you prefer. Take several natural breaths to settle into your body. Place one hand on your chest and one on your belly to help you track the vibrations.

Take a comfortable inhale through your nose, filling your lungs about 75% full—not completely full, as you need space for the sound. As you exhale, make a low, long "Voooooo" sound, like the "oo" in "book" but extended and deepened.

The sound should be low-pitched and resonate in your chest rather than your throat. You should feel vibrations in your chest cavity, and your hands should detect these vibrations. The sound doesn't need to be loud—focus on the vibration quality rather than volume.

Duration and Repetition Each Voo breath should last as long as feels comfortable—typically 10-20 seconds for the exhale. Take a natural inhale between each Voo breath, then repeat. Start with 5-10 repetitions and gradually build up to more if it feels good.

Pay attention to how your nervous system responds during and after the practice. Many people notice immediate relaxation, while others may feel temporary activation before settling into calm. Both responses are normal.

Modifications and Variations If making sound feels uncomfortable or isn't appropriate for your environment, you can practice "silent Voo"—going through the same breathing motion while imagining the sound and vibration without actually vocalizing.

You can also experiment with different pitch levels to find what feels most resonant for your body. Some people prefer a higher pitch that resonates more in the throat and head, while others find deeper tones more effective.

When to Practice Voo breath is particularly effective for:

- Releasing stress after difficult situations
- Preparing for sleep
- Discharging nervous system activation
- Times when you feel emotionally "stuck" or numb
- After exercise or physical exertion

This practice can bring up emotions or memories, which is normal and part of the healing process. If strong emotions arise, continue breathing naturally and allow whatever comes up to be present without trying to control it.

Worksheet: Personal Breath Practice Plan

Creating a personalized breathing practice ensures you have specific tools available for different situations and states. This worksheet helps you identify your patterns, preferences, and needs to develop an effective breath-based self-care routine.

Current Breathing Assessment Observe your natural breathing patterns over several days and record your findings:

Resting breathing rate (breaths per minute): _____
Primary breathing location (chest, belly, or both): _____ Breathing rhythm (regular, irregular, varies): _____ Depth of breath (shallow, moderate, deep): _____

Stress Response Patterns Notice how your breathing changes during different types of stress:

During anxiety or panic: _____ When angry or frustrated: _____ When sad or grieving: _____ During physical stress: _____ In conflict situations: _____

Technique Preferences Try each breathing exercise from this book and rate your response:

Three-dimensional breathing: How it felt: _____
Effectiveness (1-10): _____ Best time to use: _____

Coherent breathing (5-5 rhythm): How it felt: _____
Effectiveness (1-10): _____ Best time to use:
_____

Physiological sigh: How it felt: _____ Effectiveness (1-10): _____ Best time to use: _____

Extended exhale breathing: How it felt: _____
Effectiveness (1-10): _____ Best time to use:
_____

Extended inhale breathing: How it felt: _____
Effectiveness (1-10): _____ Best time to use:
_____

Voo breath: How it felt: _____ Effectiveness (1-10): _____ Best time to use: _____

Daily Practice Schedule Based on your assessment, create a realistic daily breathing practice:

Morning technique: _____ Duration: _____ Purpose: _____

Midday technique: _____ Duration: _____ Purpose: _____

Evening technique: _____ Duration: _____ Purpose: _____

As-needed techniques for: Acute stress: _____ Low energy: _____ Insomnia: _____
Anxiety: _____

Weekly Review Questions Review your practice weekly and adjust as needed:

Which techniques felt most helpful this week? _____ What situations challenged your breathing most? _____ How did regular practice affect your overall state? _____ What adjustments would improve your practice? _____

Monthly Goals Set specific, achievable goals for developing your breathing practice:

This month I want to: _____ By the end of three months: _____ Long-term breathing goals: _____

The Breathing Foundation

Conscious breathing forms the cornerstone of somatic healing work. As you develop skill with these techniques, you'll find that your breath becomes a reliable ally in navigating life's challenges. The practices in this chapter provide a foundation for the movement, touch, and sound work that follows.

Your breathing patterns reflect and influence your nervous system state moment by moment. By learning to work skillfully with your breath, you develop one of the most powerful tools available for self-regulation and healing. The techniques you've learned here will support not only your formal practice but also your ability to stay present and regulated throughout daily life.

Essential Breathing Foundations for Healing:

- Your breath provides immediate access to nervous system regulation
- Different breathing patterns create specific physiological and emotional effects
- Three-dimensional breathing restores natural, full breathing capacity

- Coherent breathing optimizes heart rate variability and nervous system balance
- The physiological sigh offers rapid stress relief in acute situations
- Extended exhale breathing calms while extended inhale breathing energizes
- Voo breath specifically stimulates vagus nerve activation for deep regulation

Chapter 5: Releasing Trauma Through Motion

Your body remembers every experience through patterns of tension, holding, and movement. Trauma often creates incomplete action patterns—frozen fight-or-flight responses that never had the chance to complete naturally. These interrupted movements remain stored in your nervous system, waiting for the opportunity to finish what they started. Movement-based healing provides that opportunity, allowing your body to complete protective responses and return to natural flow and aliveness.

Unlike exercise, which focuses on fitness goals and performance, therapeutic movement prioritizes nervous system regulation and trauma resolution. The movements that heal trauma often look nothing like conventional exercise—they might involve trembling, gentle rocking, slow reaching motions, or spontaneous gestures that arise from your body's own wisdom. Learning to trust and follow these natural impulses opens a pathway to profound healing and restoration.

Why Movement Heals

Trauma creates a fundamental disruption in your body's natural movement patterns. When faced with threat, your nervous system initiates powerful movement impulses—running away, fighting back, or pushing against restraint. If these movements can't complete due to circumstances beyond your control, the activation energy becomes trapped in your nervous system (17).

This trapped energy doesn't disappear. It continues to influence your movement patterns, emotional responses, and physical sensations years or even decades after the original event. You might find yourself feeling restless without knowing why, experiencing chronic muscle tension in specific areas, or having difficulty with certain types of movement that unconsciously remind your body of the original trauma.

Dr. David Bercier's research on trauma and movement demonstrates that completing interrupted defensive responses through conscious movement can resolve long-standing symptoms that haven't responded to other treatments (18). The key lies in following your body's natural impulses rather than imposing predetermined movements or exercises.

Consider the case of Miguel, a 29-year-old construction worker who was pinned under heavy equipment during a workplace accident. Although he escaped without serious injury, he developed chronic shoulder and neck pain that no medical treatment could resolve. He also began experiencing claustrophobia and panic attacks in confined spaces.

Through somatic movement work, Miguel discovered that his body was still trying to complete the pushing motion that had been interrupted during the accident. His shoulders and arms held tremendous tension from the thwarted attempt to push the equipment off himself. When he allowed this pushing movement to complete in a safe therapeutic setting, his chronic pain began to resolve.

Miguel learned to track the subtle sensations that preceded his panic attacks—a feeling of pressure in his chest and an urge to push outward with his arms. Instead of fighting these sensations, he learned to support them through conscious movement. He would find a wall and practice pushing against it, allowing his nervous system to complete the protective response that had been interrupted.

Over several months, Miguel's symptoms gradually diminished. His panic attacks became less frequent and less intense. His chronic pain resolved as his muscles no longer needed to hold the incomplete action pattern. Most significantly, Miguel regained confidence in his body's ability to protect him and respond appropriately to challenges.

The healing occurred not through talking about the accident or trying to understand it cognitively, but through allowing his body to complete the biological response that had been thwarted. This completion restored his nervous system's natural capacity for regulation and resilience.

The Difference Between Exercise and Therapeutic Movement

While both exercise and therapeutic movement involve physical activity, their purposes and approaches differ significantly. Exercise typically focuses on external goals—building strength, improving cardiovascular fitness, or achieving specific performance targets. Therapeutic movement prioritizes internal awareness and nervous system regulation over external achievement.

Exercise often involves:

- Predetermined movements and routines
- Focus on repetition, intensity, or duration
- Goals of improvement or progression
- Comparison with standards or other people
- Pushing through discomfort or resistance

Therapeutic movement emphasizes:

- Following internal impulses and sensations
- Attention to quality of experience rather than quantity
- Honoring your body's current capacity and needs
- Curiosity about what wants to happen naturally
- Stopping or modifying movements that create tension or overwhelm

This doesn't mean exercise can't be therapeutic or that therapeutic movement can't be vigorous. The distinction lies in the intention and awareness you bring to the activity. Running can be therapeutic if you focus on how your body feels and respond to its signals. Gentle stretching can be non-therapeutic if you force your body into positions that create tension or pain.

Lisa, a 45-year-old executive, had been a dedicated runner for years. She used running as stress relief and prided herself on maintaining consistent mileage regardless of how she felt. After developing chronic fatigue syndrome, she could no longer maintain her previous exercise routine and felt frustrated and disconnected from her body.

Lisa learned to approach movement therapeutically rather than athletically. Instead of forcing herself to run specific distances, she began each day by asking her body what kind of movement it wanted. Some days this was gentle walking; others, it was stretching or dancing to music. She learned to stop when her body felt satisfied rather than when she reached a predetermined goal.

This shift in approach helped Lisa rebuild her relationship with physical activity. She discovered that her body had been trying to communicate its needs for years, but she had been overriding these signals in pursuit of fitness goals. As she learned to listen and respond to her body's wisdom, her energy gradually returned and her enjoyment of movement was restored.

Lisa also noticed that therapeutic movement affected her emotional well-being differently than goal-oriented exercise. While running had provided stress relief through endorphin release, conscious movement helped her process emotions and develop greater body awareness. She felt more integrated and present after therapeutic movement sessions.

Finding Your Movement Style

Every person has unique movement preferences and patterns that reflect their individual nervous system, life history, and constitutional makeup. Discovering your natural movement style—the ways of moving that feel most authentic and healing for you—becomes an essential part of developing your somatic practice.

Some people are naturally drawn to flowing, dance-like movements that emphasize grace and expression. Others prefer more structured, geometric movements that engage strength and precision. Still others find healing in very subtle movements—micro-movements that might be barely visible to an observer but create significant internal shifts.

Your movement style may also vary based on your current state and needs. When feeling anxious or activated, you might need vigorous shaking or strong pushing movements. When feeling depressed or shut down, gentle swaying or reaching movements might be more appropriate. Learning to match your movement practice to your current state increases its effectiveness.

Rachel, a 38-year-old artist, initially resisted movement-based therapy because she felt awkward and self-conscious about her body. She had been told as a child that she was "clumsy" and had avoided physical activities throughout her life. The idea of moving therapeutically felt intimidating and potentially embarrassing.

Rachel's therapist suggested starting with very small movements—simply noticing how her body wanted to position itself in the chair, or allowing her hands to move freely while sitting. Rachel discovered that she was naturally drawn to spiraling, circular movements that felt fluid and organic. These movements seemed to calm her nervous system and connect her to a sense of inner flow she had never experienced.

As Rachel gained confidence, she began exploring larger movements while maintaining the circular, spiraling quality that felt authentic to her. She found that this movement style helped her access creativity and emotional expression in ways that sitting meditation or talk therapy couldn't provide. Her artwork became more expressive and alive as she developed a more connected relationship with her body.

Rachel also discovered that her "clumsiness" disappeared when she moved in ways that honored her natural patterns rather than trying to conform to external expectations. She had never been clumsy—she had simply been moving in ways that didn't match her constitutional nature.

Finding your movement style requires patience, experimentation, and willingness to look foolish. The goal isn't to move beautifully or correctly, but to discover what feels authentic and healing for your unique nervous system and body.

Exercise 5.1: Gentle Shaking for Discharge

Shaking represents one of your nervous system's most natural mechanisms for discharging excess activation and stress. Animals in the wild shake automatically after escaping from predators, allowing their nervous systems to return to baseline. Humans often suppress this natural response due to social conditioning, leading to chronic holding patterns and trapped stress energy.

This exercise reactivates your innate capacity for discharge through conscious shaking. The key is allowing the shaking to happen naturally rather than forcing it, and following your body's impulses for how fast, how long, and where to shake.

Beginning the Shake Stand with your feet about hip-width apart, knees slightly bent. Allow your arms to hang loosely at your sides. Begin by gently bouncing on the balls of your feet, letting this gentle momentum travel up through your legs into your pelvis and torso.

The movement should feel light and springy rather than jarring or forced. If you feel any discomfort in your joints, reduce the intensity or try shifting your weight from foot to foot instead of bouncing.

Allowing Natural Expansion As the bouncing continues, notice if your body wants to expand the movement. You might find that your arms want to swing, your torso wants to twist, or your head wants to move. Follow these impulses without forcing them.

Some people naturally develop a full-body shake that involves their entire system. Others prefer to keep the movement smaller and more contained. Both responses are normal and healthy—trust what feels right for your body today.

Duration and Intensity Start with 30-60 seconds of gentle shaking and gradually build up to 2-3 minutes as your body becomes accustomed to the practice. The intensity should feel manageable—energizing but not overwhelming.

Pay attention to your breathing during the shaking. Many people hold their breath when they're nervous about a new practice. Allow your breathing to stay natural and relaxed throughout the movement.

Completion and Integration When you feel ready to stop—either because you've reached your planned duration or because your body naturally wants to slow down—gradually decrease the intensity of the shaking until you're standing still.

Stand quietly for 1-2 minutes and notice any sensations, emotions, or changes in your internal state. You might feel more relaxed, energized, or emotionally moved. All responses are normal parts of the discharge process.

Modifications If standing feels unstable or uncomfortable, you can practice shaking while sitting in a chair. Focus on shaking your arms, shoulders, and upper body while keeping your feet grounded.

If you have joint problems or injuries, consult with a healthcare provider before practicing vigorous shaking. You can often modify the intensity or focus on gentler trembling movements that still provide nervous system benefits.

Exercise 5.2: Spontaneous Movement Exploration

This exercise involves following your body's natural movement impulses without predetermined goals or structures. Spontaneous movement can access and release patterns that more structured approaches might miss, allowing your nervous system to guide the healing process through its own wisdom.

The challenge for many people lies in trusting their body's impulses rather than controlling or directing the movement. This practice requires patience and willingness to look awkward or silly in service of authentic expression and release.

Creating Safe Space Find a private space where you won't be interrupted or observed. You might prefer to have music playing, but it's not necessary. Some people find that silence allows them to hear their internal rhythms more clearly.

Begin by standing, sitting, or lying down—whatever position feels most comfortable. Close your eyes and take several conscious breaths to settle into your body.

Starting with Micro-Movements Rather than jumping into large movements, begin by noticing very small impulses. Your head might want to turn slightly, your shoulders might want to shift, or your hands might want to open or close. Follow these tiny impulses without amplifying them.

This phase helps you develop sensitivity to your body's natural movement impulses before they're overridden by conscious control. Spend 2-3 minutes simply following micro-movements.

Allowing Natural Expansion As you become more attuned to your body's impulses, you might notice desires for larger movements. Your arms might want to reach, your spine might want to twist, or your whole body might want to curl up or stretch out.

Follow these impulses at their natural pace. Avoid forcing or amplifying movements, but also avoid stopping them if they want to continue. The goal is to become a responsive partner with your body's natural intelligence.

Working with Resistance You may encounter internal resistance—parts of you that feel uncomfortable with certain movements or that want to control the process. This resistance is normal and doesn't need to be overcome forcefully.

When you notice resistance, pause and acknowledge it. Sometimes simply recognizing the resistance allows it to soften. Other times, you might need to choose smaller, safer movements until your nervous system feels more comfortable with spontaneous expression.

Duration and Completion Practice for 10-20 minutes, or until you feel a natural sense of completion. Some sessions may involve vigorous movement; others might be quite subtle and internal. Both are equally valid expressions of your nervous system's current needs.

End by lying down or sitting quietly for several minutes. Notice any changes in your physical sensations, emotional state, or energy level. Allow time for integration of whatever was expressed or released during the movement.

This practice often brings up emotions, memories, or insights. Welcome whatever arises without trying to analyze or understand it immediately. Trust that your body knows how to process whatever was activated during the movement.

Exercise 5.3: Wall Push-Offs for Boundary Work

Pushing movements help activate and complete fight responses that may have been interrupted during traumatic experiences. Working with a wall provides safe resistance that allows you to practice assertiveness, boundary-setting, and self-protection in a controlled environment.

This exercise can be particularly healing for people who experienced situations where they couldn't effectively fight back or protect themselves. It helps restore the nervous system's confidence in its ability to respond to threats and assert appropriate boundaries.

Setting Up the Exercise Stand arm's length away from a solid wall. Place your palms flat against the wall at about shoulder height and shoulder-width apart. Your feet should be planted firmly on the ground, about hip-width apart.

Begin by simply leaning gently into the wall, feeling the support and resistance it provides. Notice how your body responds to having something solid to push against.

Gentle Pushing Begin pushing against the wall with moderate pressure. You're not trying to push the wall down, but rather to activate the muscles and energy of your pushing response. Focus on engaging your arms, shoulders, and core muscles.

As you push, notice what happens in your breathing, your facial expression, and your emotional state. Some people feel empowered and strong; others may feel anxious or activated. Both responses are normal.

Adding Voice (Optional) If it feels authentic and you have privacy, you can add voice to your pushing. This might be grunting sounds that naturally arise with effort, or you might experiment with saying "No!" or "Stop!" or "Get away!" if these words feel relevant to your healing process.

Adding voice can intensify the experience, so go slowly and only include it if it feels safe and appropriate. You can always practice silently and still receive significant benefits.

Varying Intensity and Pace Experiment with different intensities of pushing—from very gentle pressure to more vigorous effort. Also try different rhythms—sustained pushing, rhythmic pulses, or building and releasing pressure.

Notice which variations feel most satisfying or releasing for your nervous system. Some people prefer steady, sustained pressure; others like rhythmic pulses that allow for building and releasing energy.

Integration and Completion After 2-5 minutes of pushing (or whenever you feel complete), step back from the wall and stand quietly. Notice any changes in your posture, breathing, or internal sense of strength and capacity.

You might feel more grounded and powerful, or you might feel activated and need to discharge energy through shaking or movement. Honor whatever your system needs for integration.

Practice this exercise regularly if you struggle with boundaries, assertiveness, or feeling powerless. It can help rebuild your nervous system's confidence in its ability to protect and defend you when necessary.

Exercise 5.4: Figure-8 Flowing Movements

Figure-8 movements create integration between the right and left sides of your brain and body while promoting natural flow and rhythm. These movements can help resolve fragmentation from trauma and restore your sense of wholeness and coordination.

The infinity symbol or figure-8 pattern appears throughout nature and represents balance, integration, and continuous flow. Moving your body in these patterns can help reorganize your nervous system and promote healing integration.

Standing Figure-8s Stand comfortably with your feet about hip-width apart. Begin by tracing a horizontal figure-8 pattern in the air with one hand, keeping the movement smooth and continuous. The center crossing point should be in front of your heart area.

Focus on making the loops equal in size and maintaining a smooth, flowing rhythm. After 1-2 minutes, switch to your other hand. Then try moving both hands together in parallel figure-8s.

Notice how this movement affects your breathing, your sense of balance, and your overall energy. Many people find figure-8 movements naturally calming and integrating.

Whole-Body Figure-8s Once you're comfortable with arm movements, begin involving your whole body. Allow your spine to move in a gentle figure-8 pattern, with your pelvis leading the movement and your upper body following.

This creates a subtle undulating movement through your entire torso. Keep the movement gentle and fluid—you're not trying to create large, dramatic motions but rather to activate the natural wave-like capacity of your spine.

Walking Figure-8s If you have space, try walking in a large figure-8 pattern on the floor. This engages your whole body in the integrating movement while adding the grounding element of walking.

Walk slowly and mindfully, feeling your feet connect with the ground at each step. Allow your arms to swing naturally as you walk the figure-8 path.

Micro Figure-8s For more subtle integration, practice tiny figure-8 movements with different body parts—your eyes, tongue, shoulders, or hips. These micro-movements can be done anywhere and provide gentle nervous system integration.

Eye figure-8s can be particularly integrating. Trace a small horizontal figure-8 pattern with your eyes while keeping your head still. This activates integration between the visual and vestibular systems.

Practice figure-8 movements whenever you feel fragmented, scattered, or disconnected. They're particularly useful before important activities that require integration and coordination, or after stressful experiences that may have created internal disorganization.

Exercise 5.5: Dance Your Emotions

This exercise uses movement to express and process emotions that may be difficult to access or release through verbal methods alone. Different emotions have characteristic movement patterns, and allowing these patterns to express freely can help complete emotional cycles and restore natural flow.

Emotional expression through movement doesn't require dance training or coordination. The goal is authentic expression rather than beautiful or correct movement. Trust that your body knows how to move each emotion, even if the movements look unusual or unfamiliar.

Creating the Container Choose music that supports emotional expression, or practice in silence if you prefer. Ensure you have privacy and won't be interrupted. Give yourself permission to look silly, awkward, or dramatic—whatever wants to emerge.

Begin by standing quietly and checking in with your current emotional state. What emotions are present for you right now? You might feel multiple emotions simultaneously, or one dominant feeling.

Starting with Current Emotions Choose one emotion that's present and allow your body to begin expressing it through movement. Don't think about how the emotion should move— simply let your body respond to the feeling.

Anger might want to punch, stomp, or make sharp, staccato movements. Sadness might want to collapse, curl up, or make flowing, downward movements. Joy might want to bounce, spin, or reach upward. Trust whatever movements arise.

Exploring Stuck Emotions Sometimes emotions feel stuck or numb. If you can't access movement for a particular emotion, try starting with its physical opposite and see what happens. If you feel frozen, try small movements. If you feel scattered, try grounding movements.

You can also experiment with moving emotions you wish you could feel more fully. If you feel numb and want to access vitality, try moving joy or excitement even if you don't feel it initially. Sometimes movement can help awaken dormant emotional capacity.

Following the Movement's Evolution Allow each emotion's movement to continue until it naturally evolves or completes. You might find that expressing anger leads to sadness, or that moving sadness transforms into peace. Follow these natural progressions without forcing them.

Some emotions may want to be expressed vigorously; others may prefer subtle, internal movements. Honor the intensity level that feels authentic rather than pushing for more dramatic expression.

Integration and Completion After 10-20 minutes of emotional movement, allow yourself to slow down and come to stillness. Sit or lie down quietly and notice any changes in your emotional state, physical sensations, or energy level.

You may feel clearer, more balanced, or emotionally released. You might also feel activated and need additional time for integration. Honor whatever your system needs after emotional expression.

This practice can be particularly healing for people who were taught to suppress or control their emotions. It helps restore the natural connection between feeling and expression that supports emotional health and authenticity.

Exercise 5.6: Tension and Release Sequences

This exercise systematically creates and releases muscular tension to help discharge trapped stress and restore natural muscle tone. Many trauma survivors develop chronic muscle tension that serves as armor against perceived threats. Learning to consciously tense and release muscles can help restore your nervous system's ability to modulate between activation and relaxation.

The key to this practice lies in the contrast between tension and release. By consciously creating tension first, you can experience more complete relaxation when you let go. This teaches your nervous system that it can choose when to be activated and when to relax.

Basic Tension-Release Pattern Start by lying down or sitting comfortably. Begin with your hands—make tight fists and hold the tension for 5-10 seconds. Really squeeze and notice what it feels like to create this tension intentionally.

Then suddenly release the fists and let your hands go completely limp. Notice the contrast between the tension and the release. Feel the sensation of letting go and the relaxation that follows.

Systematic Body Progression Work through your body systematically, tensing and releasing different muscle groups:

- Arms: Tense your entire arms by making fists and pulling your arms tight against your sides, then release
- Shoulders: Scrunch your shoulders up toward your ears, then let them drop
- Face: Scrunch all your facial muscles together tightly, then let your face go soft
- Legs: Tighten your leg muscles by pressing your legs together and pointing your toes, then release
- Whole body: Tense everything simultaneously for 10 seconds, then release completely

Focusing on Problem Areas If you carry chronic tension in specific areas, spend extra time with those regions. You might tense and release your shoulders several times if you hold stress there, or work specifically with your jaw if you clench it frequently.

Sometimes areas of chronic tension resist releasing even after conscious tensing. Don't force the release—simply notice what's available and appreciate any softening that occurs.

Adding Breathing Coordinate your breathing with the tension and release cycles. Hold your breath during the tension phase, then exhale completely as you release. This adds another layer of letting go and helps deepen the relaxation response.

You can also experiment with making sounds during the release phase—sighing, groaning, or any vocal expression that wants to emerge as you let go of tension.

Completion and Integration After working through your whole body, lie quietly for 5-10 minutes and notice the overall state of your muscles and nervous system. You may feel deeply relaxed, or you might notice areas that are still holding tension.

This practice helps retrain your nervous system's relationship with tension and relaxation. Regular practice can help chronic muscle tension soften and improve your ability to relax when appropriate.

Worksheet: Movement Comfort Zone Map

Understanding your current relationship with movement helps you identify areas for growth and healing. This worksheet maps your comfort zones and challenges around different types of movement, providing guidance for developing your movement practice.

Current Movement Patterns Describe your typical daily movement:

Types of movement you do regularly: _____ How much time you spend moving each day: _____

Activities you enjoy most: _____ Activities you avoid or dislike: _____

Physical Comfort and Limitations Identify areas of comfort and challenge in your body:

Body parts that feel strong and capable: _____
Areas that feel weak, painful, or limited: _____
Movements that feel easy and natural: _____
Movements that feel awkward or difficult: _____

Emotional Responses to Movement Notice your emotional reactions to different types of movement:

Movement that makes you feel confident: _____
Movement that triggers anxiety or fear: _____
Movement that brings joy or pleasure: _____
Movement that feels emotionally neutral: _____

Social and Cultural Influences Explore how your history affects your relationship with movement:

Messages you received about your body and movement as a child: _____ Cultural or family attitudes toward physical activity: _____ Past experiences with sports, dance, or exercise: _____ Current influences on your movement choices: _____

Trauma and Movement Consider connections between trauma and movement patterns:

Types of movement that feel triggering or unsafe: _____ Body positions or movements you avoid: _____ Movements that feel protective or empowering: _____ Ways trauma may have affected your movement: _____

Movement Goals and Desires Identify what you'd like to develop:

Types of movement you'd like to try: _____
Physical capacities you'd like to build: _____
Emotional relationships with movement you'd like to change: _____ Movement practices that appeal to you: _____

Expanding Your Comfort Zone Create specific plans for gentle expansion:

One new movement to try this week: _____ One limitation you'd like to work with gradually: _____ Support you need to feel safe exploring movement: _____ Signs that indicate you're pushing too hard: _____

Weekly Movement Goals Set realistic, achievable movement goals:

Daily movement goal: _____ Weekly movement exploration: _____ Monthly movement challenge: _____ Overall movement vision: _____

Review this worksheet monthly and adjust your goals based on your developing relationship with movement. Notice how your comfort zones expand and change as you continue practicing somatic movement.

Moving Into Wholeness

Movement serves as medicine for your nervous system, offering pathways to complete interrupted responses, discharge trapped activation, and restore natural flow and aliveness. The exercises in this chapter provide starting points for developing your own movement practice, but the real healing occurs when you learn to trust and follow your body's own movement wisdom.

As you continue exploring movement, pay attention to the subtle communications from your nervous system. What movements create ease and flow? Which ones trigger defensiveness or shutdown? How does your relationship with movement reflect your relationship with life itself? These explorations prepare you for the next chapter's work with touch and boundaries—another pathway through which your body can reclaim its natural capacity for healing and connection.

Core Movement Medicine Principles:

- Trauma creates incomplete movement patterns that can be healed through conscious motion
- Therapeutic movement prioritizes internal awareness over external achievement
- Your body has natural movement preferences that reflect your unique healing needs
- Shaking, pushing, flowing, and tensing-releasing all serve different nervous system functions
- Spontaneous movement allows your body's wisdom to guide the healing process
- Movement can express and complete emotions that words cannot reach
- Regular movement practice builds nervous system resilience and integration

Chapter 6: Reclaiming Your Physical Self

Touch represents one of your most fundamental needs and one of your most vulnerable experiences. The way you were touched—or not touched—in early life shapes your nervous system's capacity for regulation, connection, and safety. Trauma often disrupts this natural relationship with touch, creating either hypersensitivity that makes contact overwhelming or numbness that disconnects you from your body's wisdom.

Healing your relationship with touch doesn't necessarily require contact with others. Self-touch and boundary work can restore your nervous system's capacity to receive comfort and protection through your own hands and awareness. Learning to touch yourself with kindness, set energetic boundaries, and sense your physical limits creates a foundation for all other healing work.

The Importance of Touch in Healing

Touch activates your parasympathetic nervous system more directly than almost any other intervention. Gentle, appropriate touch stimulates the release of oxytocin, reduces cortisol levels, and activates vagal pathways that promote calm and connection (19). For trauma survivors, however, touch can also trigger defensive responses based on past experiences of violation or harm.

The challenge lies in distinguishing between safe, healing touch and touch that recreates traumatic patterns. This distinction must be made by your nervous system, not by your rational mind. Your body holds the memory of both nurturing and harmful touch, and it will respond based on these unconscious patterns unless you consciously retrain your responses.

Research by Dr. Tiffany Field at the Touch Research Institute demonstrates that appropriate touch can improve immune function, reduce anxiety and depression, and enhance overall physical health (20). However, these benefits only occur when touch feels safe and consensual to the receiver's nervous system.

Consider the case of Angela, a 33-year-old nurse who experienced sexual trauma as a teenager. For years afterward, she avoided physical contact even with family members and romantic partners. She felt lonely and disconnected but couldn't tolerate the anxiety that touch created in her nervous system.

Angela began healing her relationship with touch through self-touch practices. She started by simply placing her own hands on her arms or shoulders while breathing consciously. Initially, even her own touch felt activating, but gradually her nervous system learned to associate gentle contact with safety and comfort.

Angela's therapist taught her to track her nervous system responses during touch. She learned to notice the difference between touch that created expansion and settling versus touch that triggered contraction and defense. This somatic discrimination allowed her to gradually expand her tolerance for safe touch.

Over time, Angela developed the capacity to receive appropriate touch from trusted friends and eventually romantic partners. The key was learning to communicate her needs clearly and stop or modify touch experiences that didn't feel safe. Her nervous system gradually learned that she had choice and control in touch interactions.

Angela's healing didn't eliminate her sensitivity to touch, but it restored her choice about when and how to engage with physical contact. She learned to honor her nervous system's protective responses while also creating opportunities for the nourishing touch her body needed.

Self-Touch as a Therapeutic Tool

Self-touch provides an ideal starting point for healing touch-related trauma because you maintain complete control over the experience. Your nervous system can learn to associate touch with safety and comfort when you're the one providing the contact. This foundation then supports your capacity to receive appropriate touch from others.

Self-touch activates the same neurological pathways as touch from others, releasing oxytocin and promoting parasympathetic activation. However, because you control every aspect of the experience, your nervous system can relax its protective vigilance and receive the benefits of physical comfort.

Many people have never learned appropriate self-touch. Cultural messages often create shame around touching your own body, particularly in nurturing rather than utilitarian ways. Learning to offer yourself comfort through touch represents a powerful act of self-care and healing.

David, a 41-year-old accountant, grew up in a family where physical affection was rare and emotional expression was discouraged. As an adult, he felt isolated and struggled with anxiety and insomnia. He had never considered that lack of nurturing touch might be contributing to his difficulties.

David learned to use self-touch as a resource for nervous system regulation. He practiced placing his hands on his heart when feeling anxious, offering himself the comfort he had never received from others. Initially, this felt awkward and unfamiliar, but gradually it became a natural source of support.

David also learned to use self-touch for sleep preparation. He would place one hand on his chest and one on his belly, feeling his breathing and offering his nervous system the security of gentle contact. This practice helped him relax and fall asleep more easily.

Over several months, David's relationship with his body transformed. He became more aware of his physical needs and more willing to offer himself comfort during difficult times. His anxiety decreased as he developed reliable self-soothing skills, and his relationships improved as he became more comfortable with his own need for comfort and connection.

The progression from self-touch to receiving touch from others occurred naturally for David. As his nervous system learned to trust touch as a source of comfort rather than threat, he became more open to appropriate physical contact with friends and romantic partners.

Boundary Work Through the Body

Your physical boundaries exist at multiple levels—your skin, your personal space, your energetic field, and your internal sense of what feels appropriate or intrusive. Trauma often damages these boundary systems, creating either rigid walls that keep everyone out or permeable barriers that offer no protection.

Healthy boundaries are semi-permeable membranes that allow nourishing contact while filtering out what feels harmful or inappropriate. They exist in the present moment and respond flexibly to current circumstances rather than being fixed based on past experiences.

Working with boundaries through your body helps restore your natural capacity to sense what feels safe and appropriate. Your nervous system provides constant feedback about proximity, touch, and interpersonal contact, but trauma can disconnect you from this internal guidance system.

Sarah, a 26-year-old social worker, struggled with boundaries in all areas of her life. She found herself agreeing to requests that felt overwhelming, staying in conversations that drained her energy, and allowing people to stand too close or touch her in ways that felt uncomfortable. She knew intellectually that she needed better boundaries but couldn't figure out how to implement them.

Sarah learned to use her body as a boundary-sensing system. She practiced noticing her physical responses when people came too close—the subtle tension in her shoulders, the urge to step back, or the feeling of her energy contracting. She learned to trust these signals as information about her boundary needs.

Sarah also practiced setting energetic boundaries through visualization and intention. She would imagine a protective bubble around her body that allowed positive energy to enter while filtering out negativity or intrusion. This mental practice helped her feel more protected in challenging social situations.

The most transformative aspect of Sarah's boundary work was learning to communicate her physical limits clearly and kindly. Instead of enduring uncomfortable situations, she learned to say things like "I need a bit more space" or "I'm not comfortable with that kind of contact." Her relationships improved as people learned to respect her needs.

Sarah discovered that healthy boundaries actually increased her capacity for intimacy rather than limiting it. When she felt protected and respected, she could open more fully to nourishing connections with others.

Exercise 6.1: Self-Holding Practices

Self-holding involves using your own hands to provide comfort, security, and nervous system regulation. These practices help you develop a nurturing relationship with your body while building your capacity to self-soothe during difficult times.

The key to effective self-holding lies in the quality of presence and intention you bring to the touch. Mechanical or distracted touch provides fewer benefits than conscious, caring contact that honors your body's need for comfort and support.

Basic Heart Hold Sit or lie comfortably and place one hand on your heart and one hand on your upper chest or throat. Feel the warmth of your hands and the gentle pressure against your body. Breathe naturally and allow your nervous system to receive the comfort being offered.

Notice how this simple contact affects your breathing, your muscle tension, and your emotional state. Many people find that heart holding creates immediate calming and a sense of being supported.

You can enhance this practice by imagining that you're offering comfort to a beloved friend or child. Bring the same quality of care and tenderness to your own body that you would offer to someone you love deeply.

Full-Body Self-Embrace Wrap your arms around yourself in a gentle, loving embrace. You might cross your arms over your chest, wrap them around your torso, or hold your own shoulders. Experiment with different positions to find what feels most comforting.

Rock gently from side to side while maintaining the self-embrace, creating the soothing motion that naturally calms nervous systems. This practice can be particularly comforting during times of grief, fear, or loneliness.

Comfort Touch for Specific Areas Place your hands on any part of your body that feels tense, painful, or in need of attention. Common areas include your forehead, the back of your neck, your lower back, or your belly. Simply rest your hands there with caring intention.

You don't need to massage or manipulate the area—simply offer the presence and warmth of your hands. Sometimes gentle circular motions feel good; other times, still contact is more soothing. Let your body guide you.

Hand-to-Hand Comfort Hold your own hands in various ways—interlacing your fingers, cradling one hand in the other, or pressing your palms together. This practice can be done discretely in public situations when you need comfort but don't want to draw attention.

Notice how different ways of holding your hands create different feelings of security and comfort. Some people prefer firm contact; others like gentle, light touch. Develop a repertoire of hand positions that feel consistently comforting.

Practice self-holding regularly, particularly during transitions, stressful periods, or times when you're feeling emotionally vulnerable. These practices help build your capacity for self-soothing and reduce dependence on others for nervous system regulation.

Exercise 6.2: Butterfly Hug for Self-Soothing

The butterfly hug, developed by Lucina Artigas for trauma survivors, provides bilateral stimulation that can help calm emotional distress and process difficult experiences. This technique combines nurturing touch with rhythmic movement to promote nervous system regulation.

The bilateral nature of this practice helps integrate right and left brain functioning while providing the comfort of self-generated touch. It's particularly useful during times of high activation, emotional overwhelm, or when processing traumatic memories.

Basic Butterfly Hug Position Cross your arms over your chest so that your hands rest on your upper arms or shoulders. Your arms should look like butterfly wings folded across your body. Ensure that your hands are positioned comfortably without creating strain in your shoulders or arms.

Close your eyes and feel the contact of your hands against your body. Notice the warmth and gentle pressure of this self-embrace. Allow your breathing to settle into its natural rhythm.

Adding Bilateral Movement Begin gently patting or stroking your arms alternately—right hand, then left hand, then right hand again. The rhythm should be slow and soothing, about one tap per second or whatever pace feels naturally calming.

Focus on the rhythmic alternation between right and left sides rather than the intensity of the touch. The movement should feel gentle and nurturing rather than vigorous or mechanical.

Coordinating with Breathing Synchronize the bilateral movement with your breathing if this feels natural. You might tap once on each inhale and once on each exhale, or develop whatever rhythm feels most soothing for your nervous system.

Some people prefer to tap continuously while breathing naturally; others like to coordinate the movement and breath more precisely. Experiment to find what works best for you.

Duration and Intensity Practice the butterfly hug for 1-3 minutes, or until you notice a shift toward greater calm or settling. The movement should feel consistently soothing—if it becomes agitating or overwhelming, slow down or pause.

You can use this technique during emotional distress, before sleep, after difficult experiences, or anytime you need self-soothing. It's particularly useful because it can be done discretely in many situations.

Variations Try different hand positions—higher or lower on your arms, firmer or lighter pressure, different rhythms of movement. Some people prefer stroking motions instead of tapping, or holding still in the butterfly position without movement.

You can also practice the butterfly hug while walking slowly, sitting in meditation, or lying down before sleep. Adapt the practice to fit different situations and needs.

Exercise 6.3: Body Boundary Visualization

This exercise helps you develop awareness of your energetic and physical boundaries while strengthening your capacity to maintain appropriate limits with others. Visualization work can help restore boundary systems that trauma may have damaged or compromised.

Strong, flexible boundaries support both intimacy and autonomy. They allow you to open fully when it's safe and appropriate while maintaining protection when needed. Boundary visualization helps train your nervous system to recognize and maintain these essential limits.

Sensing Your Current Boundaries Sit or stand comfortably and close your eyes. Begin by sensing the boundaries of your physical body—your skin as the interface between internal and external space. Notice how far your sense of "self" extends beyond your skin.

Some people sense their boundaries very close to their physical body; others feel their energy extending several feet outward.

Neither response is better—simply notice your current experience without judgment.

Pay attention to any areas where your boundaries feel particularly strong or clear, and any areas where they feel weak, missing, or confused. This information helps guide your boundary strengthening work.

Creating a Protective Boundary Imagine creating a protective boundary around yourself—this might look like a bubble of light, a protective shield, a wall of energy, or any image that represents safety and protection to you.

Experiment with different distances from your body. Some situations might require close, tight boundaries; others might allow for more expansive limits. Practice adjusting your boundary size based on your current needs.

Notice how creating this intentional boundary affects your nervous system. Many people feel immediately more relaxed and secure when they visualize clear, protective limits around their energy.

Making Boundaries Semi-Permeable Practice creating boundaries that filter rather than completely block external energy. Imagine your boundary allowing positive, supportive energy to enter while keeping out negativity, intrusion, or harm.

This might look like a mesh that filters water, a semi-permeable membrane, or a sophisticated security system that can distinguish between beneficial and harmful influences. Use whatever imagery feels most empowering for you.

Testing Boundary Strength Imagine challenging situations—someone standing too close, making inappropriate requests, or sending negative energy your way. Visualize your boundary remaining strong and clear during these tests.

Practice saying "no" or setting limits while maintaining your energetic boundary. Notice how having clear energetic limits supports your ability to communicate boundaries verbally.

Boundary Maintenance End the visualization by setting an intention to maintain your boundaries throughout the day. You might imagine checking and reinforcing your boundaries periodically, or setting up automatic boundary maintenance that doesn't require constant conscious attention.

Practice this visualization daily, particularly before entering challenging social situations or after experiences that may have compromised your boundaries. Over time, you'll develop stronger automatic boundary maintenance.

Exercise 6.4: Progressive Muscle Relaxation 2.0

This enhanced version of progressive muscle relaxation incorporates trauma-informed modifications that honor your nervous system's need for choice and control. Unlike traditional versions that might overwhelm sensitive nervous systems, this approach emphasizes titration and respect for your body's current capacity.

The practice helps you distinguish between tension and relaxation while building your capacity to consciously influence your muscle tone. For trauma survivors, developing this conscious control can help restore a sense of agency and choice in their bodies.

Preparation and Orientation Lie down or sit comfortably in a position where you feel secure and supported. Take a few minutes to orient to your environment—notice sounds, temperature, and anything else that helps your nervous system recognize current safety.

Give yourself permission to modify or stop the practice at any time. This isn't a test or performance—it's an opportunity to explore your body's capacity for relaxation while honoring your limits.

Starting with Awareness Rather than immediately creating tension, begin by simply noticing the current state of different muscle groups. Start with your feet and slowly scan through your body, observing areas of tension, relaxation, or neutrality.

This awareness phase helps you establish a baseline and ensures that you're working with your body's current reality rather than imposing predetermined expectations.

Gentle Tension Phase Choose one muscle group to work with first—perhaps your hands or feet. Create gentle tension in this area—only about 30-50% of your maximum capacity. Hold this mild tension for 3-5 seconds while breathing naturally.

The tension should feel manageable and under your control. If it creates anxiety or feels overwhelming, reduce the intensity or try a different muscle group.

Conscious Release Release the tension suddenly and completely, allowing the muscles to go limp. Focus on the contrast between tension and release, noticing the sensations of letting go.

Some areas may release completely; others might maintain some residual tension. Accept whatever level of relaxation is available rather than forcing complete release.

Working Systematically Move through your body systematically, working with one or two muscle groups at a time. Common progressions include: feet, calves, thighs, buttocks, abdomen, hands, arms, shoulders, neck, and face.

Spend extra time with areas that hold chronic tension, but don't force them to release. Sometimes awareness and gentle attention are enough to promote gradual softening.

Integration and Completion After working through your body, lie quietly for 5-10 minutes and notice the overall state of your muscles and nervous system. Some areas may feel deeply relaxed while others remain active—both responses are normal.

Set an intention to carry this awareness of tension and relaxation into your daily activities. Notice throughout the day when you're holding unnecessary tension and practice gentle release.

Exercise 6.5: Partner Exercises for Co-Regulation (Optional)

Partner work can provide powerful opportunities for healing your relationship with touch and developing capacity for co-regulation. However, this work requires significant trust and safety, and it's not appropriate for everyone or at all stages of healing.

These exercises should only be attempted with partners who understand trauma-informed consent and who can respect your boundaries completely. Never engage in partner touch work if you feel pressured or uncertain about the safety of the relationship.

Establishing Safety and Consent Before beginning any partner touch work, have detailed conversations about boundaries, consent, and safety. Discuss your trauma history to the extent that feels comfortable, and clearly communicate any touch that feels triggering or unsafe.

Establish clear signals for stopping or modifying the exercises—verbal cues like "stop" or "pause," or physical signals like raising your hand. Practice using these signals before beginning touch work to ensure they'll be honored immediately.

Basic Hand-to-Hand Contact Start with the least threatening form of touch—holding hands or placing palms together. Sit facing each other and simply make hand contact while breathing naturally and maintaining eye contact if that feels comfortable.

Notice how your nervous system responds to this contact. Does it feel calming, activating, neutral, or does the response change over time? Share your experiences verbally so your partner can learn about your nervous system responses.

Practice maintaining hand contact for several minutes while tracking your internal experience. Notice if you want more or less pressure, different hand positions, or breaks from contact.

Synchronized Breathing While maintaining hand contact, practice breathing together in the same rhythm. Start by each person breathing naturally, then gradually synchronize your breath patterns without forcing or controlling.

This practice promotes co-regulation as your nervous systems begin to entrain with each other. Many people find synchronized breathing deeply calming and connecting.

Back-to-Back Support Sit back-to-back with your partner, providing mutual support while maintaining your own boundaries. This position offers the comfort of contact without the vulnerability of face-to-face interaction.

Practice breathing together in this position, feeling the support of your partner's back while maintaining your own groundedness. This exercise can help build capacity for co-regulation while maintaining autonomy.

Setting Boundaries During Touch Practice communicating your boundary needs during partner exercises. This might involve asking for more or less pressure, different positioning, or breaks from contact.

Learning to maintain your boundaries during intimate contact is essential for healthy relationships. Use these exercises to practice clear communication about your needs and limits.

Only engage in partner touch work when it feels genuinely safe and desired. There's no rush to include others in your healing process—self-touch and boundary work provide powerful healing opportunities that don't require external relationships.

Worksheet: Boundary Assessment and Goals

Understanding your current boundary patterns helps identify areas for growth and healing. This assessment explores your boundaries in different areas of life and helps you develop specific goals for strengthening your protective and connective capacities.

Physical Boundary Assessment Evaluate your comfort with different types of physical contact:

Types of touch that feel comfortable and safe: _____ Touch that creates anxiety or discomfort: _____ How close you prefer people to stand or sit: _____ Situations where you feel your physical space is invaded: _____ Your ability to ask for more or less physical contact: _____

Emotional Boundary Assessment Explore your capacity to protect your emotional well-being:

How easily you absorb others' emotions: _____
Your ability to say no to emotional demands: _____
Situations where you feel emotionally overwhelmed by others: _____ How you protect yourself from negative emotional energy: _____ Your comfort with sharing your own emotions: _____

Energetic Boundary Assessment Notice your sensitivity to others' energy and presence:

How you feel in crowded spaces: _____ Your sensitivity to others' moods and energy: _____
Situations where you feel drained after social contact: _____ Your ability to maintain your own energy around others: _____ Practices that help you feel energetically protected: _____

Communication Boundary Assessment Assess your ability to set verbal and relational limits:

Your comfort with saying no to requests: _____
How you handle criticism or negative feedback: _____ Your ability to end conversations when needed: _____ Situations where you struggle to speak up for yourself: _____ Your skill at setting limits in relationships: _____

Boundary Violations and Patterns Identify recurring boundary challenges:

Most common types of boundary violations you experience: _____ Relationships where boundaries feel most difficult: _____ Times when you violate others' boundaries: _____ Patterns from childhood that affect current boundaries: _____ Physical symptoms that arise when boundaries are crossed: _____

Boundary Strengths and Resources Recognize your existing boundary skills and supports:

Relationships where you feel your boundaries are respected: _____ Situations where setting boundaries feels natural: _____ Skills you already have for protecting yourself: _____ People who support your boundary-setting efforts: _____ Practices that help you feel more protected: _____

Boundary Goals and Intentions Set specific, achievable goals for boundary development:

One physical boundary you want to strengthen: _____ One emotional boundary you want to develop: _____ One relationship where you need clearer boundaries: _____ One communication skill you want to practice: _____ One self-care practice that supports your boundaries: _____

Weekly Boundary Practice Create concrete steps for implementing boundary improvements:

Daily boundary awareness practice: _____ Weekly boundary challenge to work with: _____ Monthly boundary goal: _____ Support you need to maintain healthy boundaries: _____

Boundary Maintenance Strategies Develop ongoing practices for boundary health:

Warning signs that your boundaries need attention: _____ Regular practices that strengthen your boundaries: _____ People you can talk to about boundary challenges: _____ Self-care practices after boundary violations: _____

Review this assessment monthly and notice how your boundary capacity develops over time. Boundary work is ongoing—expect gradual improvement rather than dramatic overnight changes.

Reclaiming Your Physical Self

Touch and boundaries work together to help you reclaim your relationship with your physical self and your capacity for safe connection with others. The exercises in this chapter provide starting points for healing your relationship with touch while developing the boundary skills that make intimacy possible.

Your body holds the wisdom to distinguish between safe and unsafe touch, appropriate and inappropriate proximity, and nourishing versus depleting contact. Trauma may have disrupted this natural discernment, but these capacities can be restored through patient, consistent practice.

As you continue exploring touch and boundaries, trust your nervous system's responses as valid information. Your body's reactions—whether attraction, aversion, or neutral response—provide guidance about what supports your healing and what might re-traumatize. The next chapter extends this work into the healing power of sound and vibration, adding another dimension to your somatic healing toolkit.

Touch and Boundary Healing Essentials:

- Self-touch provides a safe starting point for healing touch-related trauma
- Your nervous system can learn to distinguish between safe and threatening touch
- Healthy boundaries are flexible membranes that filter rather than completely block contact

- Conscious tension and release practices restore your sense of physical agency
- Partner work requires significant safety and should never feel pressured
- Your body's responses provide reliable information about appropriate contact
- Boundary work supports both protection and intimacy in relationships

Chapter 7: Healing Through Resonance

Sound carries healing frequencies that can penetrate where touch and movement cannot reach. Every cell in your body responds to vibrational input, from the rhythm of your heartbeat to the subtle oscillations of your nervous system. Trauma often disrupts these natural rhythms, creating discord within your internal orchestra. Conscious work with sound and vibration can help restore your body's capacity for harmony and resonance.

Your voice contains particular power for healing because it emerges from within your own body, creating vibrations that massage your nervous system from the inside out. Unlike external sounds that you hear, the sounds you make activate your entire vocal apparatus—your diaphragm, ribcage, throat, and skull—creating internal massage and nervous system stimulation that promotes regulation and release.

How Sound Affects the Nervous System

Sound operates as medicine through multiple pathways in your nervous system. Specific frequencies can activate your parasympathetic nervous system, while others energize sympathetic responses. The rhythm, pitch, volume, and timbre of sound all communicate different information to your body about safety, activation, or the need for response.

Dr. Peter Levine's research demonstrates that low-frequency sounds, particularly those below 100 Hz, can directly stimulate the vagus nerve and promote nervous system regulation (21). These frequencies resonate with the natural vibrations of your internal organs and can help restore healthy autonomic function.

The auditory processing system connects directly to areas of your brain involved in emotion, memory, and arousal regulation. This explains why certain sounds can instantly transport you to different emotional states, trigger traumatic memories, or create profound calm and safety.

Consider the case of Marcus, a 34-year-old musician who developed severe performance anxiety after being humiliated during a concert. His love for music had become contaminated with fear, and he could no longer perform without experiencing panic attacks. Traditional therapy helped him understand his anxiety cognitively, but his nervous system remained activated by musical environments.

Marcus learned to use his voice as a healing instrument rather than a performance tool. He began with simple humming exercises, focusing on the internal vibrations rather than the external sound. As his nervous system learned to associate vocal expression with safety rather than judgment, his anxiety gradually decreased.

Marcus discovered that certain vocal sounds created immediate calming in his nervous system. Low, sustained tones seemed to massage his vagus nerve and promote parasympathetic activation. Higher, more energetic sounds helped him discharge anxiety and reclaim his natural enthusiasm for music.

Over several months, Marcus gradually reintroduced musical performance while maintaining his vocal healing practices. He learned to use specific vocal warm-ups that calmed his nervous system before performances, and he developed ways to stay connected to the healing aspect of sound even in evaluative situations.

Marcus's relationship with music transformed from one of fear and judgment to one of healing and authentic expression. His performances became more genuine and emotionally resonant as he learned to trust his voice as a source of regulation rather than vulnerability.

Using Your Voice for Healing

Your voice serves as both instrument and medicine, capable of creating vibrations that promote healing throughout your body. Vocal healing doesn't require singing ability or musical training—it simply requires willingness to explore sound as a tool for nervous system regulation and emotional expression.

The act of making sound activates your breathing more fully than silent breathing alone. Vocalization requires coordinated use of your diaphragm, intercostal muscles, and pelvic floor, creating internal massage and stimulation that promotes circulation and nervous system activation.

Different types of vocal sounds create different healing effects. Vowel sounds tend to resonate in specific areas of your body—"Ah" in your heart area, "Oh" in your lower belly, "Ee" in your head and throat. Consonant sounds create different types of stimulation and can help discharge stuck energy or activation.

Linda, a 47-year-old therapist, had spent years helping others process their emotions but struggled to access her own feelings. She described feeling "emotionally constipated"—aware that feelings were present but unable to move them through her system. Traditional meditation and talk therapy provided limited relief.

Linda learned to use vocal expression as a pathway to emotional release. She began with simple vowel tones, noticing how different sounds resonated in her body. She discovered that "Ah" sounds seemed to open her heart area, while "Oh" sounds helped her access sadness and grief that had been stuck for years.

Linda developed a practice of vocal expression that she used both personally and professionally. She would make different sounds while tracking her emotional state, allowing whatever wanted to be expressed to emerge through her voice. Sometimes this involved wailing or crying; other times, it was gentle humming or sighing.

The breakthrough came when Linda realized she had been trying to control and manage her emotions rather than allowing them to move through her naturally. Vocal expression taught her to trust her body's wisdom about what needed to be expressed and how.

Linda's emotional constipation gradually resolved as she learned to use her voice as a pathway for feeling and expression. Her work with clients deepened as she became more comfortable with emotional intensity in herself and others.

Vibrational Therapy Basics

Vibration affects every system in your body, from your bones and organs to your nervous system and energy field. Understanding how different types of vibration create healing effects allows you to use sound and movement more skillfully for nervous system regulation and trauma resolution.

Low-frequency vibrations (20-100 Hz) tend to resonate with your body's larger structures—bones, organs, and major muscle groups. These frequencies can help release deep tension and promote grounding and stability. Many trauma survivors find low-frequency sounds particularly soothing and regulating.

Mid-frequency vibrations (100-1000 Hz) resonate with soft tissues and can help mobilize stuck energy and emotions. These frequencies often feel energizing and can help discharge activation while maintaining a sense of safety and control.

High-frequency vibrations (above 1000 Hz) tend to resonate in your head, throat, and nervous system. They can help clear mental fog, increase alertness, and promote clarity and integration. Some people find high frequencies activating, while others experience them as uplifting and clarifying.

The key to using vibration therapeutically lies in matching the frequency to your current needs and nervous system capacity. What feels healing in one state might feel overwhelming or ineffective in another state.

James, a 52-year-old veteran, struggled with chronic pain and hypervigilance following multiple combat deployments. His nervous system remained locked in high alert, making relaxation and sleep extremely difficult. Pain medication provided limited relief and created unwanted side effects.

James learned to use specific frequencies of sound and vibration to help regulate his nervous system. He discovered that low-frequency humming seemed to calm his hypervigilance and reduce his pain levels. He developed a practice of humming specific tones while lying down, feeling the vibrations resonate through his body.

James also experimented with listening to low-frequency sound recordings—Tibetan singing bowls, didgeridoo music, and specially designed healing frequency recordings. He found that certain frequencies could shift his nervous system state within minutes, providing relief that medication hadn't been able to achieve.

The most significant discovery was that James could use his own voice to self-regulate throughout the day. When he noticed his hypervigilance increasing, he could quietly hum specific tones that helped his nervous system settle. This gave him a tool he could use anywhere without medication or external dependence.

James's pain levels decreased significantly as his nervous system learned to spend more time in regulation rather than hyperactivation. His sleep improved, and he regained capacity for activities he had avoided for years due to pain and anxiety.

Exercise 7.1: Humming for Vagus Nerve Activation

Humming creates gentle vibrations throughout your torso that can directly stimulate your vagus nerve and promote parasympathetic nervous system activation. This simple practice can be done anywhere and provides immediate nervous system regulation.

The vibrations created by humming massage your vagus nerve from within, promoting the release of calming neurotransmitters and reducing cortisol levels. Unlike external sound, humming creates vibrations that originate within your body, making it particularly effective for nervous system regulation.

Basic Humming Technique Sit or lie comfortably with your spine straight but relaxed. Close your eyes and take several conscious breaths to settle into your body. Place one hand on your chest and one hand on your throat to help you feel the vibrations.

Begin humming any pitch that feels comfortable—there's no "right" pitch for this exercise. Keep your mouth closed and allow the sound to resonate throughout your head, neck, and chest. Feel the vibrations with your hands and throughout your body.

Finding Your Resonant Pitch Experiment with different pitches to find the ones that create the most pleasant vibrations in your body. Some people prefer higher pitches that resonate in their head and throat; others find lower pitches more calming and grounding.

Notice how different pitches affect your nervous system. You might feel some pitches as calming, others as energizing, and others as neutral. Use this information to choose pitches based on your current needs.

Duration and Rhythm Continue humming for 2-5 minutes, taking breaks to breathe naturally as needed. You can hum continuously on each exhale, or create rhythmic patterns of humming and silence.

Pay attention to how your nervous system responds during and after the humming. Many people notice immediate relaxation, while others may feel temporary activation before settling into calm.

Variations and Modifications Try humming with your mouth open to create "Ahh" sounds, or experiment with different consonant sounds like "Mmm," "Nnn," or "Vvv." Each creates slightly different vibrational patterns and nervous system effects.

You can also hum silently by going through the motions without making audible sound. This still creates internal vibrations and can be used in situations where vocal expression isn't appropriate.

Integration into Daily Life Use humming as a quick nervous system reset throughout your day—before meetings, after stressful situations, or whenever you need to promote calm and centeredness. Even 30 seconds of humming can shift your nervous system state.

Exercise 7.2: Toning for Emotional Release

Toning involves using sustained vowel sounds to promote emotional expression and release. This practice can help move stuck emotions through your system while providing the nervous system regulation that comes from vocal expression.

Different vowel sounds resonate in different areas of your body and can help access and release emotions that may be stored in those regions. This makes toning particularly effective for people who struggle with emotional numbness or feeling emotionally "stuck."

Preparing for Toning Find a private space where you can make sound without feeling self-conscious or disturbing others. You might want to have tissues available, as emotional release often involves tears or other expressions.

Sit or stand comfortably and take several minutes to connect with your current emotional state. What emotions are present for you right now? What emotions feel stuck or difficult to access?

Working with Vowel Sounds Begin with the "Ah" sound, which typically resonates in your heart and chest area. Take a comfortable breath and make a long, sustained "Ahhhh" sound, allowing it to continue for as long as feels natural.

Notice how this sound affects your body and emotions. You might feel opening in your chest, emotional movement, or physical sensations. Continue with "Ah" sounds for several minutes if this feels productive.

Exploring Different Vowels Try each vowel sound and notice where it resonates in your body:

- "Ah" (as in "father") - typically resonates in the heart and chest
- "Eh" (as in "bed") - often felt in the throat and upper chest
- "Ee" (as in "see") - usually resonates in the head and throat
- "Oh" (as in "go") - commonly felt in the lower belly and pelvis
- "Oo" (as in "true") - often resonates in the lower abdomen and pelvis

Following Emotional Movement As you make different sounds, notice any emotional responses that arise. You might feel sadness, anger, joy, fear, or other emotions. Allow these feelings to be present without trying to control or change them.

Sometimes emotions want to be expressed through specific sounds—wailing for grief, growling for anger, or sighing for relief. Trust whatever sounds want to emerge and follow their natural expression.

Duration and Intensity Practice toning for 10-20 minutes, or until you feel a natural sense of completion. The intensity of sound can vary from very quiet to quite loud, depending on what feels appropriate for your emotional state.

Take breaks as needed and end the practice if it becomes overwhelming. Emotional release should feel productive rather than retraumatizing.

Integration and Aftercare After toning, sit quietly for several minutes and notice any changes in your emotional state, physical sensations, or energy level. You might feel lighter, more peaceful, or emotionally clearer.

Some people feel temporarily vulnerable after emotional release. Honor this by engaging in gentle self-care activities—drinking water, taking a bath, or spending time in nature.

Exercise 7.3: Sound Bath Creation

Creating your own sound bath involves using various sounds and instruments to create an immersive healing environment. This practice can help regulate your nervous system while exploring different types of vibrational healing.

You don't need expensive instruments to create effective sound baths. Household items, your own voice, and simple instruments can create powerful healing experiences when used with conscious intention.

Gathering Sound Sources Collect various items that can create different types of sounds:

- Singing bowls, bells, or chimes if available
- Wooden sticks, spoons, or other striking implements
- Glasses or bowls filled with water for different pitches
- Rice or beans in containers for shaking sounds
- Your own voice for toning, humming, or singing

Creating the Sound Environment Lie down comfortably in a space where you won't be disturbed. Place your sound sources within easy reach so you can access them without having to sit up or move significantly.

Begin with silence and simply listen to the ambient sounds in your environment. This helps your nervous system settle and prepares you to receive the healing sounds you'll create.

Building Layers of Sound Start with one simple sound—perhaps gentle humming or the soft ringing of a bell. Allow this sound to resonate and fade naturally before adding another layer.

Gradually build complexity by adding different sounds, rhythms, or pitches. You might alternate between vocal sounds and instrumental sounds, or combine them simultaneously.

Following Your Body's Response Pay attention to how your nervous system responds to different sounds. Notice which sounds feel calming, which feel energizing, and which feel neutral or uncomfortable.

Use this feedback to guide your sound bath creation. If a particular sound feels particularly soothing, spend more time with it. If something feels activating or uncomfortable, transition to different sounds.

Creating Rhythm and Flow Experiment with different rhythms and patterns. You might create steady, repetitive rhythms that feel grounding, or flowing, irregular patterns that feel more organic and natural.

Notice how rhythm affects your nervous system differently than pitch or timbre. Some people find steady rhythms very calming; others prefer more varied, unpredictable patterns.

Ending and Integration Gradually reduce the complexity and volume of sounds, returning to simple, single tones before ending in silence. Allow several minutes of quiet integration time to receive the benefits of the sound bath.

Notice any changes in your physical sensations, emotional state, or energy level. Many people feel deeply relaxed and restored after self-created sound baths.

Exercise 7.4: Chanting and Repetition

Chanting involves repetitive vocal expressions that can help focus your mind, regulate your nervous system, and create altered states of consciousness that support healing and integration. The repetitive nature of chanting can help quiet mental chatter while the vibrational component provides nervous system regulation.

You can use traditional chants from various spiritual traditions, or create your own repetitive sounds based on what feels healing and authentic for your system.

Simple Sound Repetition Begin with basic sound repetition using syllables like "Ma," "Om," "Ah," or "So Hum." Choose sounds that feel comfortable and pleasing to you—there's no requirement to use traditional chants if they don't resonate.

Repeat your chosen sound rhythmically, coordinating with your breathing. You might chant one syllable per exhale, or create more complex patterns that feel natural to your system.

Traditional Chant Exploration If you're interested in traditional chants, experiment with simple options like:

- "Om" or "Aum" - a universal sound representing unity
- "So Hum" - meaning "I am" in Sanskrit
- "Om Mani Padme Hum" - a Tibetan compassion mantra
- "La illaha illa'llah" - an Islamic remembrance phrase

Research the meanings of any traditional chants you use to ensure they align with your beliefs and intentions.

Creating Personal Chants Develop your own repetitive sounds based on what your body and nervous system find healing. This might be repetitive vowel sounds, meaningful words or phrases, or sounds that don't have specific meaning but feel good to make.

Some people create chants based on their healing intentions—repeating words like "peace," "strength," or "healing" in rhythmic patterns.

Duration and Rhythm Practice chanting for 5-20 minutes, finding a rhythm that feels sustainable and meditative. The pace can be slow and contemplative or more vigorous and energizing, depending on your current needs.

If your mind wanders during chanting, gently return your attention to the sound and rhythm. The repetitive nature of chanting actually supports concentration by giving your mind a simple focus point.

Group vs. Solo Practice While this is presented as a solo practice, chanting can be particularly powerful in groups where voices blend and create harmonious overtones. If you have opportunities to chant with others, notice how group resonance affects your nervous system differently than solo practice.

However, solo chanting provides the advantage of complete control over pace, volume, and content, making it ideal for trauma-sensitive individuals who need to maintain choice and agency in their healing practices.

Exercise 7.5: Music for Nervous System Regulation

Using carefully chosen music can help regulate your nervous system states and support emotional processing. Different types of music affect your autonomic nervous system in predictable ways, allowing you to consciously choose musical experiences that support your healing goals.

Understanding how rhythm, melody, harmony, and instrumentation affect your nervous system helps you curate musical experiences that promote regulation rather than dysregulation.

Assessing Current State Before choosing music, assess your current nervous system state. Are you feeling anxious and hyperactivated? Depressed and shut down? Calm but wanting more energy? Different states benefit from different types of musical support.

Notice your current breathing pattern, muscle tension, and emotional state. This baseline assessment helps you choose music that will move you toward greater regulation.

Music for Calming and Downregulation For anxiety, hyperactivation, or stress, choose music with:

- Slow tempos (60-80 beats per minute or slower)
- Simple, repetitive melodies
- Lower frequencies and deeper tones
- Minimal percussion or sudden changes
- Natural sounds like ocean waves or rain

Classical music, ambient electronic music, nature soundscapes, and traditional meditation music often provide effective downregulation.

Music for Energizing and Upregulation For depression, fatigue, or shutdown states, select music with:

- Moderate to faster tempos (100-120 beats per minute)
- Uplifting melodies and major keys
- Clear rhythmic patterns
- Energizing but not overwhelming instrumentation
- Music that inspires movement or dancing

Upbeat folk music, moderate tempo classical pieces, and energizing world music can help activate your system without creating overwhelm.

Music for Emotional Processing For accessing and processing emotions, choose music that:

- Matches or slightly amplifies your current emotional state
- Provides emotional resonance without overwhelming intensity
- Includes space for your own emotional expression
- Supports rather than suppresses whatever you're feeling

This might include melancholic music for grief processing, powerful music for anger work, or gentle music for accessing vulnerability.

Active vs. Passive Listening Experiment with both focused, active listening where music is your primary activity, and background listening where music supports other activities like movement, breathing, or meditation.

Notice how your attention affects the impact of music. Sometimes focused listening creates deeper regulation; other times, background music provides gentle support without demanding attention.

Creating Regulation Playlists Develop specific playlists for different nervous system states and needs:

- Morning activation playlist
- Stress relief playlist
- Emotional processing playlist
- Sleep preparation playlist
- Exercise/movement playlist

Update these playlists regularly as your needs and preferences change. What feels regulating in one phase of healing might feel different later in your process.

Worksheet: Personal Sound Healing Playlist

Creating a personalized sound healing collection helps you have specific tools available for different nervous system states and healing needs. This worksheet guides you through identifying and organizing sounds that support your regulation and well-being.

Current Sound Preferences Identify sounds that currently feel supportive or triggering:

Sounds that immediately calm your nervous system: _____ Sounds that feel energizing without being overwhelming: _____ Sounds that trigger anxiety or activation: _____ Sounds that feel emotionally neutral: _____ Environmental sounds that promote peace: _____

Voice and Vocal Work Assessment Explore your relationship with vocal expression:

Comfort level with making sounds or singing: _____ Vocal sounds that feel most natural to you: _____ Times when vocal expression feels healing: _____ Barriers to using your voice for healing: _____ Goals for developing vocal healing practices: _____

Instrumental and Music Preferences Identify instrumental sounds and music that support different states:

Instruments that feel particularly healing: _____ Musical genres that promote calm: _____ Music that helps you feel energized: _____ Music that supports emotional expression: _____ Music that triggers difficult emotions or memories: _____

Frequency and Vibration Responses Notice how different frequencies affect your system:

Low-frequency sounds (bass, drums, deep tones): _____ Mid-frequency sounds (guitar, piano, vocals): _____ High-frequency sounds (chimes, flutes, bells): _____ Rhythmic vs. flowing sounds: _____ Loud vs. quiet sounds: _____

State-Specific Sound Prescriptions Create sound recommendations for different needs:

When feeling anxious or activated: _____ When feeling depressed or shut down: _____ When processing grief or sadness: _____ When working with anger or frustration: _____ When wanting to feel more connected to joy: _____

Daily Sound Integration Plan how to incorporate healing sounds into your routine:

Morning sound practice: _____ Midday regulation sounds: _____ Evening wind-down sounds: _____ Background sounds for work or home: _____ Emergency regulation sounds for crisis moments: _____

Healing Sound Collection Create specific playlists or sound collections:

Nervous system calming playlist (10-15 items): _____ Energy and motivation playlist (10-15 items): _____ Emotional processing playlist (10-15 items): _____ Sleep and rest playlist (10-15 items): _____ Movement and exercise playlist (10-15 items): _____

Sound Practice Goals Set intentions for developing your sound healing practice:

Daily vocal/sound practice goal: _____ Weekly sound exploration goal: _____ Monthly sound healing challenge: _____ Long-term sound healing vision: _____

Sound Environment Optimization Consider how to create supportive sound environments:

Changes to reduce triggering sounds in your environment: _____ Sound masking strategies for noisy environments: _____ Optimal sound equipment or tools to acquire: _____ Sound healing resources to explore: _____

Update this worksheet regularly as your sound healing practice develops and your nervous system capacity changes. What feels healing may shift over time as you progress in your somatic healing journey.

Resonating with Healing

Sound and vibration offer powerful pathways for nervous system regulation and emotional healing that complement the movement, breath, and touch work of previous chapters. Your voice, in particular, provides an always-available tool for self-regulation that can be used anywhere, anytime you need nervous system support.

The healing power of sound lies not in perfect pitch or musical ability, but in your willingness to explore vocal expression as medicine and to use sound consciously for nervous system regulation. As you develop skill with these practices, you'll discover that your voice becomes a reliable ally in navigating life's challenges and supporting your ongoing healing process.

The integration practices in the next chapter will help you weave together all the somatic healing modalities you've learned—breath, movement, touch, and sound—into a comprehensive practice that supports your nervous system's natural capacity for resilience and growth.

Sound Healing Fundamentals:

- Your voice creates internal vibrations that directly stimulate nervous system regulation
- Different frequencies and rhythms affect your autonomic nervous system in predictable ways

- Humming provides immediate vagus nerve activation and parasympathetic support
- Vocal toning can help access and release stuck emotions
- Creating sound baths with simple tools provides immersive healing experiences
- Chanting and repetition calm mental activity while promoting nervous system regulation
- Carefully chosen music can support specific nervous system states and healing goals

Chapter 8: Integration Practices

Healing happens not through isolated techniques but through the gradual integration of new capacities into your daily life. The breathing, movement, touch, and sound practices you've learned become truly transformative when woven together into a coherent approach that supports your nervous system's natural rhythms and needs. Integration means learning to live somatically—making choices based on your body's wisdom rather than override patterns that may have once protected you but now limit your aliveness.

This chapter provides frameworks for combining the various somatic modalities you've explored while developing a sustainable practice that grows with you over time. The goal isn't perfection or rigid adherence to prescribed routines, but rather developing the sensitivity and skills to respond appropriately to your changing needs and circumstances.

Combining Modalities for Deeper Healing

Each somatic modality—breath, movement, touch, and sound—affects your nervous system through different pathways and offers unique healing opportunities. When skillfully combined, these approaches can create synergistic effects that surpass what any single technique can provide alone.

The art of combination lies in learning to read your nervous system's current state and choosing the modalities that will most effectively support movement toward regulation and integration. Sometimes your system needs the grounding of conscious breathing; other times, the discharge of movement or the comfort of self-touch.

Dr. Pat Ogden's research in Sensorimotor Psychotherapy demonstrates that combining somatic modalities can help reorganize traumatic responses more effectively than single-modality approaches (22). The key lies in sequencing different interventions based on your nervous system's capacity and current needs.

Consider the case of Samantha, a 39-year-old emergency room doctor who struggled with chronic hyperactivation from years of high-stress work. Single modality approaches provided temporary relief, but her nervous system would quickly return to its habitual state of hypervigilance.

Samantha learned to create sequences that addressed different aspects of her stress response. She would begin with conscious breathing to establish basic regulation, then use movement to discharge excess activation, followed by self-touch for comfort and sound work for deeper nervous system integration.

The sequence typically started with coherent breathing to shift her from sympathetic dominance toward parasympathetic activation. Next, she would practice gentle shaking or spontaneous movement to discharge the accumulated stress energy from her workday. After movement, she would use self-holding practices to provide comfort and security. Finally, she would end with humming or toning to promote deep vagal activation and integration.

This multi-modal approach helped Samantha's nervous system learn new patterns of regulation that persisted longer than single-technique interventions. Her chronic hyperactivation gradually gave way to a more flexible nervous system that could activate when needed and relax when appropriate.

The key breakthrough was learning to customize her practice based on her current state rather than following a rigid routine. Some days she needed more movement; others required extended breathing work. Her practice became a dialogue with her nervous system rather than an imposed structure.

Creating Your Personal Practice

Developing a sustainable personal practice requires balancing structure with flexibility, consistency with adaptation to changing needs. Your practice should feel supportive rather than burdensome, healing rather than effortful, and authentic to your unique nervous system and life circumstances.

Effective somatic practices typically include daily maintenance elements that support baseline regulation, plus targeted interventions for specific challenges or goals. The maintenance elements help prevent overwhelm and build nervous system resilience, while targeted practices address particular symptoms or areas of growth.

Your practice will likely change as your healing progresses. What serves you in early recovery may feel too simple or constraining later. What challenges you today may become effortless tomorrow. Building flexibility into your practice structure allows for this natural progression.

Robert, a 44-year-old teacher recovering from a divorce, initially needed extensive daily practices to manage his anxiety and depression. His early practice included 20 minutes of breathing work, 15 minutes of movement, and 10 minutes of sound work each morning, plus additional interventions throughout the day as needed.

As Robert's nervous system stabilized, his daily practice gradually simplified to 10 minutes of integrated work that combined breathing, gentle movement, and vocal expression. However, he maintained the capacity to expand his practice during stressful periods or when facing particular challenges.

Robert learned to think of his practice as a toolkit rather than a prescription. His basic daily practice provided maintenance and prevention, while his expanded practices served as medicine for acute stress or growth opportunities. This flexibility prevented his practice from becoming rigid or burdensome.

The most important aspect of Robert's practice development was learning to listen to his body's guidance about what was needed each day. Sometimes his nervous system called for vigorous movement; other times it needed gentle stillness. His practice became increasingly responsive to his authentic needs rather than externally imposed expectations.

Robert also discovered that his practice naturally evolved through different phases—periods of intensive work during challenging life transitions, maintenance phases during stable times, and integration periods when new capacities were becoming effortless parts of his daily functioning.

Working with Resistance and Obstacles

Resistance to somatic practices often arises from protective parts of your nervous system that fear change, even positive change. These obstacles aren't character flaws or signs of insufficient motivation—they're natural expressions of your system's attempts to maintain familiar patterns that once served important protective functions.

Common forms of resistance include forgetting to practice, feeling too busy for self-care, experiencing increased symptoms when beginning new practices, or feeling that the work is too slow or ineffective. Each type of resistance provides information about your nervous system's current capacity and protective strategies.

Rather than fighting resistance, effective somatic work involves developing curiosity about what your resistance is trying to protect. Sometimes resistance signals that you're moving too fast or pushing too hard. Other times, it reflects old patterns that need gentle updating rather than forceful override.

Maria, a 35-year-old social worker, consistently forgot to do her breathing practices despite intellectually understanding their importance. She felt frustrated with herself and interpreted her forgetfulness as lack of commitment to her healing.

Exploration revealed that Maria's resistance stemmed from childhood experiences where self-care was viewed as selfish. Her nervous system associated taking time for herself with danger and disapproval. Her forgetting was actually a protective mechanism designed to keep her safe from perceived judgment.

Maria addressed her resistance by starting with extremely small practices—one conscious breath at a time rather than 10-minute sessions. She also worked on developing self-compassion around her self-care efforts, recognizing that resistance was a normal part of changing deeply ingrained patterns.

As Maria's nervous system gradually learned that self-care was safe, her resistance naturally decreased. She found herself remembering her practices more often and feeling less guilty about taking time for her own well-being.

Maria also learned to view resistance as valuable information rather than something to overcome. When resistance increased, she would explore whether she was pushing too hard, whether external stressors required adjustments to her practice, or whether new areas of healing were ready to be addressed.

Exercise 8.1: Morning Somatic Ritual

Creating a morning somatic practice helps establish nervous system regulation before encountering the day's challenges. This ritual sets the tone for how your nervous system will respond to stress, opportunities, and interactions throughout the day.

Your morning practice should be sustainable for your current life circumstances—it's better to do five minutes consistently than to plan twenty minutes that you'll skip when life gets busy. The goal is establishing a regular check-in with your nervous system that provides foundation for the day ahead.

Assessment and Orientation (2-3 minutes) Begin by sitting quietly and assessing your current state. Notice your breathing pattern, energy level, emotional state, and any physical sensations that draw your attention.

Ask yourself: "What does my nervous system need this morning?" You might need calming if you wake up anxious, energizing if you feel sluggish, or grounding if you feel scattered.

Take a moment to orient to your environment—notice sounds, temperature, lighting, and anything else that helps your nervous system recognize current safety and resources.

Breathing Foundation (3-5 minutes) Choose a breathing practice based on your current needs:

- Coherent breathing (5-5 rhythm) for general regulation
- Extended exhale breathing if you feel anxious or activated
- Extended inhale breathing if you feel tired or depressed
- Three-dimensional breathing to establish full breathing capacity

Allow your breathing to establish a foundation of regulation that will support your day's activities.

Movement Integration (3-5 minutes) Add gentle movement that feels appropriate for your current state:

- Gentle stretching or yoga poses
- Figure-8 flowing movements for integration
- Shaking or bouncing for energy and discharge

- Spontaneous movement following your body's impulses

Let your movement support whatever shift your nervous system is making from sleep to wakefulness.

Touch and Boundaries (1-2 minutes) Include brief self-touch practices:

- Heart hold for comfort and connection
- Self-embrace for security
- Boundary visualization for protection
- Any self-touch that feels nurturing

Sound and Voice (1-2 minutes) Complete with vocal expression:

- Humming for vagal activation
- Toning vowel sounds
- Sighing or yawning to complete the wake-up process
- Any sounds that want to emerge naturally

Intention Setting (1 minute) End by setting an intention for your day—not a goal to achieve, but a quality of being you want to cultivate. This might be presence, kindness, flexibility, or any quality that feels supportive.

Adapt this structure based on your available time and current needs. The key is creating a consistent practice that helps your nervous system transition from sleep to active engagement with life.

Exercise 8.2: Evening Discharge Practice

Evening practices help your nervous system process and integrate the day's experiences while preparing for restorative sleep. This practice emphasizes discharge and release rather than activation, helping your system transition from day consciousness to sleep preparation.

Many people struggle with sleep because their nervous systems remain activated by the day's stresses. Creating an intentional transition practice helps signal to your body that it's safe to relax and restore.

Daily Review and Acknowledgment (2-3 minutes) Begin by acknowledging your day without judgment—both challenges you navigated and positive experiences you enjoyed. This helps your nervous system recognize completion rather than carrying unfinished stress into sleep.

Notice any areas of your body that feel tense or activated from the day's activities. Common areas include shoulders, jaw, stomach, and lower back.

Activation Discharge (5-10 minutes) Release accumulated stress through movement:

- Gentle shaking to discharge nervous system activation
- Tension and release sequences for chronically tight areas
- Spontaneous movement to express whatever your body needs to release
- Any movement that helps stress energy move through and out of your system

The goal is to help incomplete stress responses finish and discharge rather than remaining stored in your nervous system overnight.

Emotional Expression (3-5 minutes) Use sound to process emotional residue from the day:

- Sighing or yawning to release stress
- Toning or humming to promote regulation

- Any vocal expression that helps emotions move through your system
- Silent sound work if vocal expression isn't appropriate

Transition to Rest (5-10 minutes) Shift toward sleep preparation:

- Extended exhale breathing to activate parasympathetic nervous system
- Progressive muscle relaxation to release physical tension
- Self-holding practices for comfort and security
- Gentle, slow movements that promote settling

Sleep Preparation (2-3 minutes) Complete with practices that specifically support sleep:

- Body scan meditation
- Gratitude practice to promote positive nervous system states
- Visualization of your safe space
- Any ritual that signals to your nervous system that it's time to rest

This practice helps create clear transition from day activities to sleep preparation, giving your nervous system permission to release the day's stress and enter restorative states.

Exercise 8.3: SOS Emergency Regulation Sequence

Having a reliable sequence for acute stress or overwhelm provides your nervous system with immediate support during crisis moments. This practice should be simple enough to remember under stress and effective enough to create noticeable regulation within a few minutes.

The SOS sequence combines the most immediately effective techniques from each modality to provide rapid nervous system support when you need it most.

Immediate Safety and Grounding (30 seconds)

- Feel your feet on the ground and your body in the chair or space
- Orient to your environment by naming three things you can see, hear, and feel
- Remind yourself "I am safe right now" or whatever phrase feels authentic

Breathing Regulation (1-2 minutes)

- Use the physiological sigh (double inhale, long exhale) 3-5 times
- If still activated, continue with extended exhale breathing
- If feeling shut down, use gentle extended inhale breathing

Physical Regulation (1-2 minutes)

- Self-holding practices—hand on heart, self-embrace, or butterfly hug
- Gentle movement if space allows—rocking, swaying, or foot tapping
- Progressive muscle relaxation if you're sitting or lying down

Vocal Regulation (30-60 seconds)

- Humming quietly (can be done silently if necessary)
- Sighing or yawning to activate parasympathetic nervous system
- Any vocal sound that feels regulating

Integration and Assessment (30 seconds)

- Notice any changes in your nervous system state
- Assess whether you need additional support or professional help
- Plan your next steps from a more regulated state

Practice this sequence when you're calm so it becomes automatic during stress. Modify it based on your environment—you can do most elements discretely in public settings.

The goal isn't to eliminate all stress or activation, but to help your nervous system return to your window of tolerance where you can think clearly and respond appropriately.

Exercise 8.4: Weekly Integration Session

Weekly longer practices provide opportunities for deeper work and integration that daily practices may not accommodate. These sessions allow time for more extensive exploration and processing of whatever is arising in your healing journey.

Weekly sessions also provide space for trying new techniques, deepening familiar practices, and addressing specific challenges or areas of growth that require more time and attention.

Extended Check-In (5-10 minutes) Begin with a thorough assessment of your current state and week:

- How has your nervous system been functioning this week?
- What challenges have you faced? What successes have you experienced?
- What areas of your body, emotions, or relationships need attention?
- What aspects of your healing journey want exploration today?

Targeted Practice Selection (20-40 minutes) Choose practices based on your current needs:

- If you've been stressed: Extended relaxation and discharge practices
- If you've been shut down: Energizing and activation practices
- If you've been emotionally numb: Expression and movement practices
- If you've been overwhelmed: Grounding and containment practices

Allow more time than daily practices permit for full exploration and integration of whatever arises.

Integration and Processing (10-15 minutes) End with integration practices:

- Journaling about insights, experiences, or shifts you notice
- Art, drawing, or other creative expression of your internal experience
- Quiet meditation or reflection on your growth and healing process
- Setting intentions for the coming week based on what you've learned

Resource Building (5 minutes) Update your resource library based on the week's experiences:

- What practices felt most helpful this week?
- What new resources or supports did you discover?
- What practices need modification or weren't as effective?
- What do you want to explore or develop further?

These longer sessions help consolidate the gains from your daily practices while providing space for deeper exploration and healing work.

Exercise 8.5: Body-Based Problem Solving

This practice uses your body's wisdom to approach decisions and challenges from a somatic perspective rather than relying solely on mental analysis. Your nervous system often contains information about situations that your rational mind hasn't yet recognized.

Body-based decision making doesn't replace rational analysis but adds another layer of information that can guide you toward choices that support your overall well-being and authentic growth.

Problem or Decision Identification Choose a specific issue you're facing—this might be a relationship decision, work challenge, health concern, or any situation where you're feeling stuck or uncertain.

Frame the issue as clearly as possible while remaining open to new perspectives that might emerge through the somatic exploration.

Baseline State Assessment Before exploring the specific issue, establish awareness of your current nervous system state. Notice your breathing, muscle tension, energy level, and emotional state as neutrally as possible.

This baseline helps you distinguish between your general state and responses that are specifically related to the issue you're exploring.

Option Exploration Through the Body If you're facing a decision between specific options, explore each possibility through your body:

- Imagine choosing Option A and notice your body's response
- Pay attention to expansion/contraction, energy changes, breathing shifts
- Imagine choosing Option B and notice any differences in your somatic response
- Continue with additional options if relevant

Scenario Visualization For more complex problems, visualize different scenarios and track your nervous system responses:

- Imagine the situation continuing as it is—how does your body respond?
- Visualize potential changes or interventions—what feels expansive or contractive?
- Explore various approaches to the challenge through your body's wisdom

Integration and Action Planning After exploring through your body, integrate somatic information with rational analysis:

- What did your body tell you about different options or approaches?
- How does this somatic information complement or challenge your mental analysis?
- What actions feel most aligned with both your body's wisdom and rational thinking?
- What next steps support both your nervous system needs and practical requirements?

This practice helps develop trust in your body's guidance while maintaining integration with cognitive problem-solving abilities.

Worksheet: Personalized Practice Schedule

Creating a realistic, sustainable practice schedule ensures that somatic healing becomes integrated into your daily life rather than remaining an additional burden or obligation.

Current Life Assessment Honestly evaluate your current schedule and capacity:

Available time for morning practice: _____
Available time for evening practice: _____
Available time for weekly longer sessions: _____
Days of the week that feel most supportive for practice: _____ Times of day when you feel most motivated for self-care: _____

Energy and Motivation Patterns Notice when you naturally have energy for different types of practices:

Times when you feel motivated for physical practices: _____ Times when you prefer quiet, internal practices: _____ Days when you typically feel more or less capacity: _____ Seasonal patterns that affect your practice motivation: _____ Life situations that increase or decrease your practice consistency: _____

Practice Preferences and Effectiveness Based on your experience with different practices:

Most effective practices for your anxiety/activation: _____ Most effective practices for depression/shutdown: _____ Practices you find most enjoyable and sustainable: _____ Practices that feel most challenging but beneficial: _____
Practices you want to develop more skill with: _____

Daily Practice Design Create a realistic daily routine:

Morning routine (duration and specific practices): _____ Midday check-ins or brief practices: _____ Evening routine (duration and specific practices): _____ Emergency/SOS practices for acute stress: _____ Minimum practice you can maintain during busy periods: _____

Weekly Practice Planning Design weekly rhythm:

One longer practice session per week: _____ Day and time that works best for extended practice: _____ Weekly review and practice planning time: _____ Integration activities (journaling, creative expression): _____ Social or community aspects of practice: _____

Monthly and Seasonal Adaptations Plan for natural variations:

Monthly practice review and adjustment schedule: _____ Seasonal modifications to your practice: _____ Adaptations for high-stress periods: _____ Expansions during stable periods with more capacity: _____ Annual retreat or intensive practice periods: _____

Obstacle Prevention and Management Prepare for common challenges:

Most likely obstacles to consistent practice: _____ Strategies for maintaining practice during busy periods: _____ Support systems for accountability and motivation: _____ Modifications for illness, travel, or disrupted routines: _____ Signs that your practice needs adjustment or professional support: _____

Progress Tracking and Celebration Create systems for acknowledging growth:

How you'll track progress and changes: _____
Weekly or monthly celebration of your practice commitment: _____ Markers of nervous system improvement to notice: _____ Ways to acknowledge small gains and improvements: _____ Annual review of your somatic healing journey: _____

Review and adjust this schedule monthly, recognizing that your practice will naturally evolve as your healing progresses and life circumstances change.

Weaving the Threads of Healing

Integration represents the ultimate goal of somatic healing work—not the mastery of individual techniques, but the development of a lived relationship with your body's wisdom that informs how you move through the world. As you continue practicing the exercises and approaches in this workbook, you're developing capacities that extend far beyond symptom management to encompass a fundamental transformation in how you experience yourself and engage with life.

The practices you've learned provide a foundation, but your body's wisdom will guide you toward the specific combinations and modifications that serve your unique healing journey. Trust this internal guidance as much as you trust the structured exercises. Your nervous system knows what it needs to heal—these practices simply provide tools for listening to and supporting that natural wisdom.

The journey ahead involves continued integration of these somatic capacities into all areas of your life. The next chapters will explore how to apply these skills to specific trauma patterns, relationships, and long-term sustainable living. Your foundation in somatic healing practices prepares you for this more advanced work of living from your body's wisdom rather than despite it.

Integration Practice Essentials:

- Combining modalities creates synergistic healing effects beyond single approaches
- Personal practice develops through dialogue with your nervous system's changing needs
- Resistance provides valuable information about your system's protective strategies
- Daily rituals establish baseline regulation while targeted practices address specific challenges
- Emergency sequences provide immediate support during acute stress or overwhelm
- Weekly sessions allow deeper exploration and integration of healing themes
- Body-based decision making adds somatic wisdom to rational problem-solving

Chapter 9: Targeted Healing Approaches

Different types of trauma create distinct patterns in your nervous system, each requiring specialized approaches for effective healing. A car accident leaves different imprints than childhood neglect, just as cultural oppression creates unique adaptations compared to medical trauma. Understanding these specific patterns allows you to choose healing approaches that address the particular ways trauma has organized itself in your body and nervous system.

This chapter explores four major categories of trauma patterns and provides targeted interventions for each. Rather than using generic approaches for all trauma responses, you'll learn to recognize the specific signatures of different trauma types and apply healing strategies that match your nervous system's particular adaptations.

Developmental Trauma Adaptations

Developmental trauma occurs during critical periods of brain and nervous system development, typically before age six. Unlike single-incident traumas, developmental trauma involves ongoing patterns of inadequate care, emotional neglect, abuse, or family dysfunction that shape how your nervous system learns to function in the world (23).

Children who experience developmental trauma must adapt their nervous systems to survive in unpredictable or threatening environments. These adaptations become deeply embedded patterns that persist into adulthood, affecting attachment, emotional regulation, self-sense, and interpersonal relationships.

Common developmental trauma adaptations include hypervigilance, emotional numbness, difficulty trusting others, challenges with self-soothing, and a fragmented sense of self. These patterns developed as survival strategies but often limit adult functioning and relationships.

Consider the case of Elena, a 42-year-old therapist who struggled with perfectionism, people-pleasing, and chronic anxiety despite years of traditional therapy. Her childhood involved emotionally volatile parents who alternated between neglect and criticism, creating an environment where she never felt safe or securely attached.

Elena's nervous system had adapted to this environment by developing exquisite sensitivity to others' moods combined with a chronic state of hypervigilance. She could sense subtle changes in people's emotions before they were consciously aware of them, but this same sensitivity left her feeling overwhelmed and exhausted in most social situations.

Elena's healing work focused on helping her nervous system distinguish between past danger and present safety. She learned to recognize when her hypervigilance was responding to current threats versus reacting to old patterns of family unpredictability.

Through somatic work, Elena discovered that her perfectionism served as a protective strategy—if she could be perfect, maybe she could avoid the criticism and rejection she had experienced as a child. Her body held this perfectionism as chronic muscle tension, particularly in her shoulders and jaw.

Elena's healing involved learning to relax these protective holdings while developing new ways to feel safe in relationships. She practiced allowing imperfection in small ways, tracking how her nervous system responded when she made mistakes or received feedback.

Over time, Elena's chronic anxiety decreased as her nervous system learned that current relationships didn't carry the same dangers as her childhood environment. Her perfectionism softened into healthy standards, and her sensitivity to others became a gift rather than a burden.

The key breakthrough was helping Elena understand that her survival adaptations had been brilliant responses to a difficult situation. Rather than pathologizing her patterns, she learned to appreciate the creativity of her childhood nervous system while updating these strategies for her current adult life.

Shock Trauma Responses

Shock trauma results from overwhelming single incidents that exceed your nervous system's capacity to cope and integrate the experience. Car accidents, natural disasters, medical emergencies, assault, or witnessing violence can create shock trauma responses that remain active in your nervous system long after the event has ended (24).

Unlike developmental trauma, shock trauma often involves specific triggers, flashbacks, and body memories related to the original incident. Your nervous system remains prepared to respond to similar threats, creating symptoms like hyperstartle, avoidance, intrusive memories, and panic responses.

Shock trauma typically involves incomplete defensive responses—fight, flight, or freeze reactions that couldn't complete during the original event. Healing often requires helping these responses finish in a safe therapeutic environment.

Consider the case of Marcus, a 35-year-old firefighter who developed PTSD after being trapped in a building collapse. Despite years of dangerous work, this particular incident overwhelmed his nervous system's capacity to cope. He began experiencing panic attacks, insomnia, and an inability to return to firefighting work.

Marcus's body held the memory of being pinned and unable to move during the collapse. His nervous system remained in a chronic state of freeze, alternating with periods of hyperactivation when triggered by reminders of the incident.

Marcus's healing work focused on helping his nervous system complete the interrupted defensive responses from the building collapse. Through careful titration, he learned to reconnect with the fighting and struggling impulses that had been suppressed during the incident.

Marcus practiced pushing movements against walls, allowing his body to complete the struggle response that had been thwarted when he was trapped. He also worked with breathing exercises that helped discharge the hyperactivation that accumulated during the freeze response.

The breakthrough came when Marcus's body was able to complete the sequence of responses that had been interrupted during the collapse—struggling, then escaping, then discharging the activation through trembling and deep breathing.

As Marcus's nervous system completed these interrupted responses, his panic attacks decreased and his sleep improved. He was eventually able to return to firefighting work, though he developed better awareness of his nervous system limits and self-care needs.

Marcus's healing demonstrated that shock trauma often requires completing biological responses rather than just understanding the incident cognitively. His body needed to finish what it had started during the collapse before his nervous system could return to normal functioning.

Complex PTSD Considerations

Complex PTSD develops from repeated trauma exposure over extended periods, particularly in situations where escape isn't possible. This might include childhood abuse, domestic violence, captivity, or ongoing oppression. Complex PTSD creates more pervasive symptoms than single-incident trauma, affecting identity, relationships, and fundamental sense of safety in the world (25).

Complex PTSD often involves emotional dysregulation, negative self-concept, interpersonal difficulties, dissociation, and loss of meaning or hope. These symptoms reflect the ways your nervous system adapts to chronic threat and helplessness.

Healing complex PTSD requires addressing both specific traumatic incidents and the overall impact on your nervous system's development and functioning. This often involves longer-term therapy and multiple healing modalities.

Consider the case of Sarah, a 44-year-old nurse who experienced sexual abuse by multiple family members throughout her childhood and adolescence. The abuse was accompanied by threats and manipulation that prevented her from seeking help or escaping the situation.

Sarah developed complex PTSD symptoms including severe dissociation, emotional numbness, difficulty trusting others, and a fragmented sense of self. She described feeling like "a collection of parts" rather than an integrated person.

Sarah's healing work needed to address both the specific abuse incidents and the overall impact on her nervous system development. She worked with parts of herself that held different aspects of her experience—the part that survived by disconnecting, the part that held anger, the part that maintained hope.

Sarah's somatic work focused on helping her develop a sense of integrated embodiment. She learned to track sensations in her body, which had been largely inaccessible due to chronic dissociation. She practiced grounding techniques that helped her stay present rather than disconnecting during stress.

The process was slow and required careful attention to Sarah's capacity. Sometimes working with body awareness triggered dissociation, so her therapist taught her to titrate the work—spending short periods in body awareness followed by grounding and stabilization.

Sarah's healing involved rebuilding basic trust in her body's signals and her ability to protect herself. She learned to recognize the early signs of dissociation and use grounding techniques to stay present during challenging situations.

Over several years, Sarah developed greater integration between her different parts and improved capacity for staying present in her body. Her relationships became more authentic as she learned to trust her own perceptions and communicate her needs clearly.

Sarah's case illustrates that complex PTSD healing often requires longer timelines and more extensive support than single-incident trauma recovery. The healing addresses not just specific events but fundamental patterns of nervous system organization.

Cultural and Collective Trauma

Cultural and collective trauma affects entire communities or groups, transmitted through families, social systems, and cultural practices. This includes historical trauma from slavery, genocide, war, or oppression, as well as ongoing systemic trauma from discrimination, poverty, or cultural displacement (26).

Cultural trauma often involves inherited nervous system patterns passed through epigenetic mechanisms and family systems. Children may carry trauma responses to events they didn't directly experience but that affected their family or community.

Healing cultural trauma requires addressing both individual symptoms and the larger social context that created and maintains traumatic conditions. This often involves connecting with cultural resources, community healing, and social justice efforts.

Consider the case of David, a 38-year-old teacher whose grandparents survived the Holocaust. Despite never experiencing war directly, David struggled with chronic anxiety, hypervigilance, and difficulty feeling safe in the world. His family rarely discussed their history, but the trauma lived in unspoken fears and protective behaviors.

David's nervous system carried patterns of hypervigilance and mistrust that seemed disproportionate to his actual life experiences. He found himself constantly scanning for threats and had difficulty relaxing even in safe environments.

David's healing work involved understanding how trauma can be transmitted across generations through family patterns, nervous system adaptations, and epigenetic changes. He learned that his anxiety wasn't just personal but connected to his family's survival strategies.

David worked to distinguish between inherited trauma responses and current reality. He practiced grounding techniques that helped his nervous system recognize present-moment safety rather than responding to historical threats that no longer existed.

David also connected with other descendants of Holocaust survivors, finding community support and understanding that reduced his sense of isolation. He learned about his family's history in ways that honored their survival while freeing him from carrying their trauma patterns.

Through somatic work, David learned to discharge inherited activation while honoring the strength and resilience that also came through his family line. He developed practices that helped him stay present rather than living in inherited fear patterns.

David's healing included connecting with cultural practices and community rituals that supported collective healing. He found that individual therapy was most effective when combined with community connection and cultural reclamation.

His case demonstrates that cultural trauma healing often requires both individual nervous system work and community-based approaches that address the social context of trauma.

Exercise 9.1: Inner Child Body Dialogue

This exercise helps you connect with and heal younger parts of yourself that may be carrying unresolved trauma. Your inner child often holds trauma in specific body locations, and establishing dialogue through the body can provide healing that traditional inner child work sometimes misses.

The practice involves identifying body areas that seem to hold young energy or trauma, then establishing gentle communication with these parts through sensation, movement, and imagery.

Preparation and Settling Find a comfortable position where you feel safe and won't be interrupted. Close your eyes and take several minutes to settle into your body using breath awareness and grounding techniques.

Set an intention to approach any young parts of yourself with kindness, curiosity, and patience. These parts may be shy, scared, or protective, and they need to feel safe before opening to dialogue.

Body Scanning for Young Energy Slowly scan through your body, paying attention to areas that feel particularly vulnerable, protected, or young. These might be areas of chronic tension, numbness, or places that draw your attention for unclear reasons.

Common areas where inner child energy concentrates include the belly, heart, throat, and pelvis. However, your inner child might be located anywhere in your body, so scan without preconceptions.

Initial Contact and Acknowledgment When you identify an area that seems to hold young energy, place your hands there gently and simply acknowledge this part of yourself. You might say internally: "I notice you there" or "I see you" or simply offer your presence.

Notice how this part responds to your attention. Does it seem to welcome contact, shrink away, or remain neutral? Respect whatever response you receive without trying to force connection.

Gentle Inquiry and Listening Ask this part of yourself simple questions and listen for responses through sensation, imagery, emotion, or intuitive knowing:

- How old do you feel?
- What do you need right now?
- What do you want me to know?
- How can I help you feel safer?

Responses might come as words, images, sensations, emotions, or just subtle shifts in the area you're focusing on. Trust whatever you receive, even if it doesn't seem logical.

Offering Comfort and Resources Based on what this part communicates, offer appropriate comfort. This might involve:

- Gentle self-touch or holding
- Breathing warmth and love into the area
- Visualizing surrounding this part with protection
- Making promises about current safety or future care

Only offer what you can genuinely provide. Your inner child needs authentic reassurance rather than empty promises.

Integration and Ongoing Connection End the session by expressing appreciation to this part of yourself and making a commitment to ongoing connection. This might involve:

- Daily check-ins with this part
- Specific self-care practices this part requested
- Changes in how you treat yourself or make decisions
- Professional support if this part needs more healing than you can provide

Practice this exercise regularly, building relationship with different parts of yourself over time. Inner child healing often requires ongoing attention rather than single sessions.

Exercise 9.2: Releasing Hypervigilance Patterns

Hypervigilance involves your nervous system remaining constantly alert for threats, even in safe environments. This pattern often develops as protection against repeated danger but becomes exhausting when maintained chronically in safe situations.

This exercise helps retrain your nervous system to distinguish between genuine threats and old patterns of hypervigilance, gradually building capacity for relaxation and trust.

Hypervigilance Assessment Begin by identifying your personal hypervigilance patterns:

- What does your body do when scanning for threats?
- Which senses become heightened when you're hypervigilant?
- How does hypervigilance affect your breathing, muscle tension, and posture?
- What triggers typically activate your hypervigilance?

Spend several minutes consciously engaging your hypervigilance patterns. Notice how your eyes move, how your breathing changes, how your muscles organize for quick response.

Conscious Safety Assessment Practice deliberately assessing your current environment for actual threats:

- Look around your space systematically, noting actual safety indicators
- Listen for sounds that indicate current safety versus danger
- Notice temperature, lighting, and other environmental factors
- Assess the actual probability of threat in your current situation

This conscious assessment helps your rational mind provide evidence of safety to your hypervigilant nervous system.

Gradual Hypervigilance Release Once you've consciously assessed your safety, begin gradually releasing hypervigilance patterns:

Eye Softening: Allow your eyes to soften their focus rather than maintaining sharp, scanning awareness. Practice peripheral vision and gentle gazing rather than vigilant watching.

Breath Settling: Shift from shallow, quick breathing to deeper, slower rhythms. Use extended exhale breathing to signal safety to your nervous system.

Muscle Releasing: Consciously relax muscles that organize for quick escape or defense—particularly shoulders, jaw, and legs. Use progressive muscle relaxation to release hypervigilant muscle tension.

Nervous System Downregulation: Practice techniques that specifically calm your sympathetic nervous system—humming, gentle movement, or coherent breathing.

Building Trust in Safety Develop practices that help your nervous system learn to trust safety:

- Spend time in environments that feel genuinely safe
- Practice relaxation in gradually more challenging situations
- Build relationships with people who feel consistently safe
- Develop environmental modifications that support your sense of safety

Hypervigilance Titration When you need to be appropriately alert (driving, walking alone at night), practice conscious hypervigilance that you can turn on and off:

- Deliberately activate appropriate alertness for genuinely risky situations
- Practice returning to relaxation when the situation no longer requires vigilance
- Build flexibility between alert and relaxed states rather than chronic hypervigilance

This helps you maintain appropriate caution without exhausting hypervigilance patterns.

Exercise 9.3: Reconnecting After Dissociation

Dissociation involves disconnecting from your body, emotions, or present-moment awareness as protection against overwhelming experiences. While dissociation can be protective during trauma, chronic disconnection limits your capacity for full engagement with life.

This exercise provides gentle techniques for reconnecting with your body and present-moment awareness while respecting your nervous system's need for protection.

Recognizing Dissociation Learn to identify your personal dissociation patterns:

- Physical signs: numbness, feeling disconnected from body, spatial disorientation
- Emotional signs: feeling detached, emotions seeming distant or unreal
- Cognitive signs: difficulty concentrating, feeling like you're watching yourself from outside
- Temporal signs: losing time, feeling like things aren't quite real

Practice recognizing these signs early, before dissociation becomes complete disconnection.

Grounding Through the Senses Use sensory experiences to reconnect with present-moment reality:

5-4-3-2-1 Technique: Identify 5 things you can see, 4 things you can touch, 3 things you can hear, 2 things you can smell, 1 thing you can taste.

Temperature Awareness: Notice the temperature of air on your skin, hold something warm or cool, splash cool water on your face.

Texture Exploration: Touch different textures around you—smooth, rough, soft, hard—to reconnect with physical sensation.

Movement and Position: Feel your body's weight and position, move different body parts to reestablish body awareness.

Gentle Body Reconnection Gradually reconnect with your body without forcing or rushing:

Breathing Awareness: Focus on the physical sensations of breathing—air moving in and out, chest and belly movement.

Heartbeat Connection: Place your hand on your heart and feel its rhythm, using this as an anchor to your physical presence.

Progressive Body Contact: Starting with less vulnerable areas like hands or feet, gradually reestablish connection with your whole body.

Movement Integration: Use gentle movement to help reconnect with your body—swaying, stretching, or walking slowly.

Emotional Reconnection Carefully reconnect with emotions while maintaining safety:

- Start with neutral emotions before approaching more intense feelings
- Use emotional vocabulary to name what you're experiencing
- Practice feeling emotions in your body rather than just thinking about them
- Build tolerance for emotional intensity gradually

Managing Reconnection Overwhelm Sometimes reconnection can feel overwhelming. Develop strategies for titrating the process:

- Take breaks from reconnection work when needed
- Practice pendulation between connection and protection
- Use grounding techniques if reconnection becomes too intense
- Seek professional support if dissociation is severe or chronic

Exercise 9.4: Anger Discharge Sequences

Anger often becomes stuck in your nervous system when it couldn't be expressed safely during traumatic experiences. This trapped anger can create chronic tension, depression, or explosive outbursts that seem disproportionate to current situations.

This exercise provides safe ways to discharge stored anger energy while building your capacity to feel and express anger appropriately in current relationships.

Anger Assessment and Preparation Before working with anger, assess your current relationship with this emotion:

- How comfortable are you with feeling angry?
- What messages did you receive about anger in your family?
- How does anger typically show up in your body?
- What triggers tend to activate your anger?

Create a safe space for anger work where you won't be interrupted and can make noise if needed. Have water available and plan for integration time after the practice.

Physical Anger Expression Use movement and sound to safely discharge anger energy:

Pillow Hitting: Use pillows or cushions to punch, hit, or throw safely. Focus on the physical discharge rather than imagining specific people or situations.

Stomping and Kicking: Stomp your feet or kick (safely into the air or against cushions) to activate the fighting energy that anger contains.

Vocal Expression: Make angry sounds—growling, yelling, or saying "NO!" loudly. This helps discharge anger through your voice and throat.

Pushing and Pulling: Use isometric exercises—pushing against walls or pulling on towels—to activate the muscular energy of anger.

Anger Boundary Work Practice using anger energy for healthy boundary setting:

- Practice saying "NO!" with conviction and power
- Use angry energy to push away imagined violations
- Practice protective stances and movements
- Experiment with taking up space when angry

This helps you channel anger into protective rather than destructive directions.

Anger and Grief Integration Often anger covers hurt, disappointment, or grief. After discharging anger energy, explore what other emotions might be present:

- Notice if sadness, hurt, or fear emerges after anger expression
- Allow these more vulnerable emotions to be present
- Use self-comfort techniques for any grief or hurt that arises

- Practice holding both anger and vulnerability simultaneously

Anger in Relationship Practice expressing anger in ways that maintain connection:

- Use "I" statements to express angry feelings
- Practice expressing anger without attacking or blaming
- Learn to express anger while staying open to the other person's response
- Build capacity for conflict without disconnection

This helps you use anger as information about your needs and boundaries rather than as a weapon against others.

Exercise 9.5: Grief Movement Rituals

Grief often becomes stuck in your body when it couldn't be fully expressed during loss or trauma. This trapped grief can create numbness, chronic sadness, or difficulty experiencing joy and connection.

This exercise uses movement and ritual to help grief move through your system naturally, honoring losses while restoring your capacity for joy and connection.

Grief Preparation and Intention Before working with grief, set clear intentions and create appropriate support:

- Identify specific losses you want to honor (people, relationships, dreams, innocence)
- Create sacred space with meaningful objects, photos, or symbols
- Plan for integration and self-care after grief work
- Have tissues and comfort items available

Begin by acknowledging the courage it takes to feel grief and the love that grief represents.

Embodied Grief Expression Allow grief to move through your body naturally:

Flowing Movements: Let your body move like water—flowing, curving, melting movements that match grief's fluid nature.

Contracting and Expanding: Practice movements that mirror grief's rhythm—curling inward with pain, opening outward with love and memory.

Reaching and Releasing: Reach toward what you've lost, then practice letting go through releasing movements.

Earth Connection: Lie on the ground or floor, allowing gravity to hold you while you feel your grief.

Vocal Grief Expression Use sound to move grief through your system:

- Wailing, crying, or keening sounds
- Singing songs that connect you to your loss
- Speaking to your lost loved one or lost aspects of yourself
- Using foreign language sounds that express grief beyond words

Grief Rituals and Ceremony Create meaningful rituals that honor your losses:

- Write letters to what you've lost and read them aloud
- Create art, poetry, or music that expresses your grief
- Plant something or create a memorial space
- Share stories about your loss with trusted others

Grief and Gratitude Integration Practice holding grief and gratitude simultaneously:

- Express gratitude for what the loss brought to your life
- Appreciate your capacity to love deeply enough to grieve
- Honor both the pain of loss and the gift of having loved
- Find ways to carry forward the positive aspects of what you've lost

Completing Grief Cycles Learn to complete grief cycles rather than getting stuck:

- Allow grief to move through your body without stopping it
- Practice returning to life and joy after grief expression
- Build tolerance for feeling grief without being overwhelmed by it
- Develop rituals for honoring anniversary dates and grief triggers

Worksheet: Trauma Pattern Identification

Understanding your specific trauma patterns helps you choose targeted healing approaches rather than generic trauma treatments. This worksheet guides you through identifying the particular ways trauma has organized in your nervous system.

Trauma History Assessment Identify the types of trauma you've experienced:

Developmental/childhood trauma (abuse, neglect, family dysfunction): _____ Shock trauma (accidents, violence, medical emergencies): _____
Complex/repeated trauma (ongoing abuse, war, captivity): _____ Cultural/collective trauma (discrimination, historical trauma, systemic oppression): _____

Medical trauma (invasive procedures, life-threatening illness): _____

Nervous System Pattern Recognition Identify your dominant nervous system responses:

Hyperactivation patterns (anxiety, hypervigilance, panic): _____ Hypoactivation patterns (depression, numbness, disconnection): _____ Mixed patterns (alternating between activation and shutdown): _____ Dissociation patterns (feeling unreal, disconnected, lost time): _____ Fragmentation patterns (feeling like different parts of yourself): _____

Body-Based Trauma Signatures Notice how trauma shows up in your body:

Areas of chronic tension or pain: _____ Areas of numbness or disconnection: _____ Movement patterns you avoid or struggle with: _____
Breathing patterns related to trauma: _____ Posture or positioning that feels protective: _____

Trigger Pattern Analysis Identify your specific trauma triggers:

Environmental triggers (sounds, smells, places): _____ Interpersonal triggers (conflict, authority, intimacy): _____ Internal triggers (emotions, sensations, memories): _____ Temporal triggers (anniversaries, seasons, times of day): _____
Somatic triggers (body positions, touch, movement): _____

Emotional Pattern Recognition Notice your trauma-related emotional patterns:

Emotions you feel too much (anger, fear, sadness): _____ Emotions you struggle to access (joy, anger, grief): _____ Emotions that feel dangerous or overwhelming: _____ Emotional patterns in relationships: _____ Emotional regulation strategies you use: _____

Protective Strategy Assessment Identify how you've adapted to protect yourself:

People-pleasing or conflict avoidance: _____
Hypervigilance or control patterns: _____ Isolation or relationship avoidance: _____ Perfectionism or overachievement: _____ Addictive or compulsive behaviors: _____

Healing Priority Identification Based on your pattern analysis, identify healing priorities:

Most urgent trauma pattern to address: _____ Body areas needing the most attention: _____ Nervous system capacities you want to develop: _____
Emotions you want to work with: _____
Relationships patterns you want to change: _____

Resource and Capacity Assessment Evaluate your current healing resources:

Internal resources (strengths, coping skills, positive memories): _____ External resources (supportive people, safe places, healing activities): _____ Professional resources (therapists, healers, medical support): _____ Areas where you need additional support: _____ Current capacity for trauma work: _____

Targeted Healing Plan Create specific healing approaches for your patterns:

Daily practices for your nervous system patterns: _____ Weekly exercises for your specific trauma type: _____ Professional support needed for your healing: _____ Environmental changes that would support your healing: _____ Long-term healing goals based on your trauma patterns: _____

Update this assessment every few months as your healing progresses and new patterns become apparent or old patterns resolve.

Addressing Your Unique Healing Path

Trauma creates unique patterns in each nervous system, requiring individualized approaches for effective healing. The exercises and concepts in this chapter provide starting points for working with different trauma types, but your own nervous system will guide you toward the specific combinations and modifications that serve your healing journey.

Understanding your particular trauma patterns allows you to choose targeted approaches rather than hoping generic techniques will address your specific needs. As you continue practicing these exercises, pay attention to which approaches feel most healing and which patterns in your nervous system respond most readily to different interventions.

The next chapter explores how these individual healing capacities support and are supported by healing in relationship with others. Your growing nervous system resilience prepares you for the more complex work of maintaining your healing while navigating intimate connections with other people.

Core Trauma Pattern Healing Principles:

- Different trauma types create distinct nervous system adaptations requiring specific approaches
- Developmental trauma affects attachment and requires patient rebuilding of basic safety
- Shock trauma involves completing interrupted defensive responses through body-based work
- Complex PTSD requires addressing both specific incidents and overall nervous system patterns
- Cultural trauma healing includes both individual work and community connection
- Inner child work through the body accesses healing that cognitive approaches may miss
- Hypervigilance, dissociation, anger, and grief each require specialized discharge techniques

Chapter 10: Somatic Healing with Others

Your nervous system developed in relationship and continues to heal in relationship. While individual somatic practices provide essential tools for self-regulation, the deeper healing of trauma often requires safe connection with others. Your capacity to co-regulate with trusted people, communicate your needs clearly, and maintain your boundaries while staying open to connection represents the ultimate expression of nervous system health.

This chapter explores how to apply somatic awareness to your relationships, using your body's wisdom to navigate the complex terrain of human connection. You'll learn to recognize when relationships support or dysregulate your nervous system, develop skills for healthy co-regulation, and practice maintaining your individual healing while engaging authentically with others.

The Neurobiology of Connection

Human beings are biologically designed for connection. Your nervous system regulates more easily in the presence of calm, safe others than it does in isolation. This capacity for co-regulation begins in infancy when caregivers help regulate your emotional states, and it continues throughout your life as a source of healing and resilience (27).

However, trauma can disrupt your natural capacity for co-regulation, creating protective patterns that interfere with healthy connection. You might find yourself either too dependent on others for regulation or too independent to receive the support that relationships can provide.

Dr. Stephen Porges' Polyvagal Theory explains that your nervous system constantly evaluates the safety of social interactions through a process called neuroception—unconscious detection of cues that signal safety or danger in relationships (28). Learning to track these subtle social cues helps you choose relationships that support your healing.

Consider the case of Jennifer, a 36-year-old marketing executive who struggled with intimate relationships despite being socially successful. She could maintain friendships and work relationships effectively, but romantic intimacy triggered intense anxiety and a desire to flee.

Jennifer's nervous system had learned early that emotional closeness led to unpredictability and potential hurt. Her mother struggled with depression and would alternate between emotional engulfment and cold withdrawal. Jennifer's young nervous system adapted by maintaining distance from deep emotional connection.

As an adult, Jennifer found herself attracted to partners but unable to tolerate the vulnerability that intimate relationships required. Her nervous system would activate whenever relationships moved beyond surface-level connection, triggering fight-or-flight responses that drove her to create distance.

Jennifer's healing work focused on helping her nervous system learn to distinguish between past relational dangers and current safety. She practiced staying present during moments of activation in her relationship, using breathing and grounding techniques to maintain connection with her partner rather than automatically fleeing.

Jennifer learned to communicate her nervous system needs to her partner rather than managing her anxiety alone. She would say things like "I'm feeling activated right now and need a few minutes to ground myself" rather than creating emotional distance without explanation.

Over time, Jennifer's capacity for intimacy gradually expanded. Her nervous system learned that current relationships didn't carry the same unpredictability as her childhood experiences. She developed the ability to use co-regulation with her partner rather than relying solely on self-regulation.

The breakthrough came when Jennifer realized that her partner's calm presence actually helped regulate her nervous system when she allowed it. Instead of seeing her partner's support as weakness or dependence, she learned to receive co-regulation as a natural part of healthy relationship.

Co-regulation vs. Self-regulation

Both self-regulation and co-regulation play essential roles in nervous system health. Self-regulation involves your individual capacity to manage your emotional states, stress responses, and activation levels. Co-regulation involves the mutual influence that occurs when two or more nervous systems interact to support each other's optimal functioning.

Healthy adults need both capacities. Self-regulation provides independence and resilience when you're alone or when others aren't available for support. Co-regulation offers the additional nervous system resources that come from safe connection with others.

Trauma can disrupt the balance between these capacities, creating either excessive dependence on others (under-developed self-regulation) or excessive independence (inability to co-regulate). Healing often involves developing whichever capacity is less available while maintaining the strengths you already have.

Consider the case of Robert, a 48-year-old therapist who prided himself on his self-regulation skills. He could manage stress, maintain emotional equilibrium, and help others regulate their nervous systems. However, he struggled to receive support from others and felt uncomfortable when people tried to comfort or help him.

Robert's childhood involved taking care of an alcoholic parent and providing emotional support for his younger siblings. His nervous system learned to be the regulator for others but never experienced reliable co-regulation from caregivers.

As an adult, Robert found intimate relationships challenging because he couldn't allow others to support him during difficult times. His automatic response to stress was to withdraw and self-regulate rather than reach out for connection and co-regulation.

Robert's healing work involved learning to receive co-regulation without feeling weak or burdensome. He practiced asking for support during minor stresses before building up to bigger challenges. He learned to track how his nervous system responded when others offered comfort.

Robert discovered that receiving co-regulation actually enhanced rather than diminished his self-regulation capacity. When he allowed others to support him, he felt more resourced and capable rather than depleted or dependent.

The process required Robert to challenge deeply held beliefs about strength and independence. He learned that interdependence—the ability to both give and receive support—represented greater maturity than independence alone.

Robert's relationships deepened as he became more able to receive care from others. His professional work also improved as he developed greater empathy for clients who struggled with receiving support.

Healing Attachment Through the Body

Attachment patterns formed in early relationships create templates for how your nervous system expects to be treated in intimate connections. Secure attachment develops when caregivers consistently respond to your needs with sensitivity and reliability. Insecure attachment patterns emerge when caregivers are inconsistent, absent, or harmful.

These early patterns become encoded in your nervous system and continue to influence your adult relationships. However, attachment patterns can be modified through new experiences of safe, responsive connection—a process called earned security (29).

Somatic approaches to attachment healing focus on helping your nervous system learn new patterns of connection through body-based experiences rather than relying solely on cognitive understanding of attachment dynamics.

Consider the case of Maria, a 41-year-old teacher who struggled with an anxious attachment style. She found herself constantly worried about her partner's feelings toward her, seeking excessive reassurance, and feeling devastated by any signs of disconnection or conflict.

Maria's early attachment experiences involved a loving but anxious mother who was often overwhelmed by life stresses. Maria learned to monitor her mother's emotional state carefully and to feel responsible for maintaining her mother's emotional equilibrium.

As an adult, Maria's nervous system remained hypervigilant to signs of relationship threat. She could detect subtle changes in her partner's mood or energy before her partner was consciously aware of them, but this sensitivity created chronic anxiety about relationship security.

Maria's healing work involved learning to distinguish between her own emotional state and her partner's. She practiced grounding techniques that helped her stay connected to her own nervous system rather than becoming completely attuned to her partner's state.

Maria learned to use her body as a resource for relationship security rather than constantly seeking external reassurance. She practiced feeling her feet on the ground during relationship anxiety, using her breathing to self-soothe, and offering herself comfort through self-touch.

The transformation occurred gradually as Maria's nervous system learned that relationship security came from her own internal resources combined with her partner's consistent responsiveness. She became less reactive to her partner's normal mood variations and more able to communicate her needs directly.

Maria's relationships became more authentic as she stopped managing her anxiety through people-pleasing and started expressing her genuine thoughts and feelings. Her partner appreciated the reduction in anxiety and the increased authenticity in their connection.

Exercise 10.1: Eye Contact Titration

Eye contact represents one of the most direct forms of nervous system communication between people. For many trauma survivors, sustained eye contact can feel threatening or overwhelming, while lack of eye contact can create disconnection and misunderstanding.

This exercise helps you build tolerance for appropriate eye contact while maintaining choice and control over the level of connection that feels safe.

Preparation and Safety Practice this exercise with someone you trust—a friend, family member, or romantic partner who understands your healing process. Establish clear agreements about respecting boundaries and stopping whenever either person feels uncomfortable.

Begin by sitting comfortably facing each other at a distance that feels manageable. You should be close enough to see each other clearly but far enough apart that you don't feel crowded or threatened.

Baseline Assessment Before beginning formal eye contact work, assess your current capacity:

- How does eye contact typically feel for you?
- What happens in your nervous system when you make eye contact?
- What messages did you receive about eye contact in your family?
- How long can you maintain comfortable eye contact currently?

Share these observations with your partner so they understand your starting point and can support your process appropriately.

Gradual Eye Contact Building Start with very brief periods of eye contact—just 2-3 seconds—followed by looking away or closing your eyes. Notice your nervous system response to even this brief connection.

Gradually increase the duration of eye contact as your comfort allows. Some people can progress to 30 seconds or longer; others may find 10 seconds quite challenging. Honor your own pace rather than forcing yourself to match external expectations.

Pay attention to the quality of eye contact as well as duration. Soft, open gazing feels different than intense staring. Practice different qualities of eye contact to find what feels most comfortable and connecting.

Working with Activation If eye contact triggers anxiety, activation, or other difficult responses:

- Use breathing techniques to stay present during mild activation
- Practice grounding through your body while maintaining eye contact
- Take breaks to regulate your nervous system before continuing
- Communicate your experience to your partner rather than managing alone

Building Connection Through Eyes As your tolerance for eye contact increases, experiment with different types of connection:

- Practice giving and receiving compassion through eye contact
- Use eye contact to communicate without words
- Notice how sustained eye contact affects your sense of being seen and accepted
- Explore maintaining eye contact during difficult conversations

Integration into Daily Life Apply your growing eye contact capacity to everyday relationships:

- Practice appropriate eye contact with service providers, colleagues, and acquaintances
- Notice how eye contact affects your professional and social interactions
- Use eye contact skills to enhance intimacy in close relationships
- Develop flexibility in eye contact based on cultural and situational appropriateness

Exercise 10.2: Synchronized Breathing

Breathing together creates one of the most direct forms of nervous system co-regulation. When two people synchronize their breathing patterns, their nervous systems begin to entrain with each other, promoting mutual calm and connection.

This exercise teaches you to co-regulate through conscious breathing while maintaining your individual nervous system awareness and boundaries.

Partner Preparation Choose a partner with whom you feel safe and comfortable. This might be a romantic partner, close friend, family member, or healing partner. Both people should consent enthusiastically to the practice and feel free to stop at any time.

Discuss any breathing difficulties, trauma related to breathing, or other concerns before beginning. Establish signals for stopping or modifying the practice if either person becomes uncomfortable.

Positioning and Initial Connection Sit facing each other at a comfortable distance, or lie down side by side if that feels more relaxing. Close your eyes or maintain soft eye contact, whichever feels more comfortable for both people.

Spend several minutes breathing naturally without trying to synchronize. Simply notice your own breathing pattern and become aware of your partner's breathing rhythm without trying to change either pattern.

Finding Natural Synchronization Often, breathing will begin to synchronize naturally without effort as your nervous systems attune to each other. Notice if this spontaneous synchronization occurs and how it feels for both of you.

If natural synchronization doesn't occur, begin gently adjusting your breathing rhythm to match your partner's, or work together to find a mutual rhythm that feels comfortable for both people.

Exploring Different Breathing Patterns Once you establish comfortable synchronized breathing, experiment with different patterns:

- Coherent breathing (5 seconds in, 5 seconds out) for nervous system balance
- Extended exhale breathing for calming and relaxation
- Energizing breathing patterns for increased vitality
- Three-dimensional breathing for full capacity and aliveness

Notice how different breathing patterns affect both your individual state and the quality of connection between you.

Adding Sound and Vibration If both people feel comfortable, add vocal sounds to your synchronized breathing:

- Humming together on the exhale
- Making "Ah" sounds or other vowel tones
- Chanting simple sounds or mantras
- Creating improvised vocal harmony

The vibrational component adds another layer of nervous system connection and can deepen the co-regulating effects of synchronized breathing.

Integration and Completion End the practice by returning to natural, individual breathing patterns. Spend several minutes sitting quietly together, noticing any changes in your individual nervous system state and the quality of connection between you.

Discuss your experiences openly, sharing what felt supportive, challenging, or surprising about the practice. This communication helps build trust and understanding for future co-regulation exercises.

Exercise 10.3: Safe Touch Exploration

Touch represents one of the most powerful forms of co-regulation, but it can also trigger strong defensive responses in trauma survivors. This exercise provides a framework for exploring appropriate touch in ways that honor both people's boundaries and nervous system needs.

This practice should only be attempted with partners who feel completely safe and trustworthy. Any hesitation or uncertainty about safety indicates that touch work should be postponed until greater trust and safety are established.

Consent and Boundary Setting Before any physical contact, have detailed conversations about consent, boundaries, and expectations:

- Discuss your individual comfort levels with different types of touch
- Establish clear signals for wanting more, less, or different touch
- Agree on specific types of touch that feel appropriate to explore
- Create agreements about respecting "no" immediately without question or negotiation

Both people should feel enthusiastic about participating rather than accommodating the other person's desires.

Starting with Minimal Touch Begin with the least threatening forms of touch—perhaps holding hands or placing one hand on the other person's shoulder. Even these simple touches can provide significant co-regulating benefits.

Spend several minutes with minimal touch, tracking both your own nervous system response and staying attuned to your partner's experience. Notice how even light touch affects your breathing, muscle tension, and emotional state.

Gradual Touch Expansion If minimal touch feels comfortable and beneficial, gradually explore slightly more extensive contact:

- Hand placement on non-threatening areas like arms, hands, or shoulders
- Back-to-back contact while sitting together
- Side-by-side contact while lying down
- Appropriate embrace or holding

Move very slowly and check in frequently about comfort levels. The goal is building positive associations with safe touch rather than pushing through discomfort.

Communication During Touch Maintain verbal communication throughout touch exploration:

- Share what feels good, comforting, or supportive
- Communicate immediately about any discomfort or activation
- Ask for specific modifications rather than enduring uncomfortable touch
- Express appreciation for touch that feels healing or connecting

This communication builds trust and helps both people learn about helpful versus unhelpful touch.

Working with Touch Triggers If touch triggers difficult responses, work with these reactions rather than avoiding them:

- Use breathing and grounding techniques to stay present during mild activation
- Practice communicating about triggered responses without completely disconnecting
- Modify touch intensity, location, or style to find what feels manageable
- Take breaks for individual regulation before returning to touch exploration

Integration and Aftercare After touch exploration, spend time integrating the experience:

- Notice any changes in your nervous system state from the touch
- Discuss what felt most and least comfortable about the experience
- Plan appropriate self-care for any emotions or sensations that arose
- Appreciate the courage both people showed in exploring vulnerable connection

Exercise 10.4: Conflict Resolution Through Body Awareness

Conflict often triggers protective responses that interfere with effective communication and problem-solving. This exercise teaches you to use somatic awareness to stay present and connected during disagreements while maintaining your boundaries and authentic expression.

Learning to navigate conflict from an embodied place rather than reactive protective patterns can transform relationships and create opportunities for deeper intimacy and understanding.

Pre-Conflict Preparation Before addressing specific conflicts, build skills for staying present during activation:

- Practice individual regulation techniques until they become readily accessible
- Develop awareness of your personal conflict triggers and patterns
- Learn to recognize early signs of nervous system activation during disagreements
- Establish agreements with your partner about how to handle activation during conflict

Both people should practice these skills individually before attempting conflict resolution together.

Somatic Awareness During Conflict When conflict arises, maintain attention to your nervous system state while engaging with the disagreement:

Breathing Awareness: Notice if your breathing becomes shallow, rapid, or restricted during conflict. Use conscious breathing to maintain nervous system regulation while discussing difficult topics.

Body Position: Pay attention to your posture and positioning. Are you leaning forward aggressively, pulling back defensively, or maintaining open, grounded positioning?

Muscle Tension: Track areas where you hold tension during conflict—jaw, shoulders, stomach. Use brief muscle releases to maintain physical openness during disagreement.

Emotional Tracking: Notice emotions as they arise in your body rather than being swept away by them. This helps you communicate about your feelings rather than acting them out.

Regulated Communication Strategies Practice communication approaches that maintain nervous system regulation:

- Use "I" statements to express your experience rather than attacking your partner
- Take breaks when activation becomes too intense for productive communication
- Ask for specific changes rather than making global criticisms
- Listen to your partner's perspective while maintaining connection to your own needs

Working with Activation During Conflict When you notice nervous system activation during conflict:

- Acknowledge your activation to your partner rather than hiding it
- Use brief grounding or breathing techniques to return to your window of tolerance
- Ask for the time or space you need to regulate before continuing the conversation
- Practice returning to the conflict discussion after regulation rather than avoiding resolution

Co-Regulation During Conflict Learn to use connection with your partner to support mutual regulation during disagreement:

- Maintain appropriate eye contact during difficult conversations
- Use touch if both people find it helpful during conflict (hand-holding, appropriate embrace)
- Practice synchronized breathing to promote mutual calm during heated discussions
- Remember your care for each other even while disageing about specific issues

Conflict Resolution and Integration Complete conflict resolution with integration practices:

- Appreciate both people's willingness to work through difficult issues
- Acknowledge any nervous system activation that occurred and provide mutual support
- Celebrate successful regulation and communication during the conflict
- Plan follow-up conversations if the issue requires ongoing attention

Worksheet: Relationship Somatic Patterns

Understanding how your nervous system responds in different relationships helps you choose connections that support your healing while addressing patterns that might interfere with healthy intimacy.

Relationship Nervous System Assessment Notice how your nervous system responds in different types of relationships:

With romantic partners: _____ With family members: _____ With close friends: _____ With work colleagues: _____ With authority figures: _____ With new acquaintances: _____

Activation Triggers in Relationships Identify specific interpersonal triggers:

Behaviors from others that activate your nervous system: _____ Types of conversations that feel threatening: _____ Relationship situations that trigger fight/flight/freeze: _____ Conflicts or disagreements that feel overwhelming: _____ Intimacy levels that create anxiety or shutdown: _____

Co-Regulation Patterns Assess your capacity for healthy co-regulation:

People whose presence naturally calms your nervous system: _____ Relationships where you can both give and receive support: _____ Your comfort level with depending on others: _____ Your ability to provide co-regulation for others: _____ Situations where co-regulation becomes codependency: _____

Communication and Boundaries Evaluate your relationship communication patterns:

Your ability to express needs clearly: _____ Your comfort with saying no in relationships: _____ How you handle conflict and disagreement: _____ Your capacity to maintain boundaries while staying connected: _____ Areas where you tend to people-please or accommodate: _____

Attachment and Connection Patterns Notice your attachment-related patterns:

How you respond when people get close to you: _____ Your comfort level with emotional intimacy: _____ Patterns of pursuing or distancing in relationships: _____ Your ability to trust others with vulnerability: _____ How you handle relationship endings or loss: _____

Touch and Physical Connection Assess your relationship with touch in relationships:

Your comfort level with appropriate touch: _____
Types of touch that feel supportive vs. threatening: _____ Your ability to ask for physical comfort when needed: _____ How you navigate physical

boundaries: _____ Changes in touch needs based on your nervous system state: _____

Relationship Healing Goals Identify specific relationship patterns you want to change:

One relationship skill you want to develop: _____
One boundary pattern you want to strengthen: _____ One communication pattern you want to improve: _____ One co-regulation capacity you want to build: _____ One relationship fear you want to work with: _____

Support and Resource Planning Plan support for your relationship healing:

Professional support needed for relationship issues: _____ Friends or family who can support your relationship growth: _____ Self-care practices that support your relationship capacity: _____
Relationship education or training that would be helpful: _____ Community or group support for relationship healing: _____

Relationship Practice Planning Create specific practices for relationship healing:

Daily practices that support your relationship capacity: _____ Weekly relationship practices to try with safe partners: _____ Monthly relationship goals and assessments: _____ Communication skills to practice in low-stakes relationships: _____
Boundary practices to implement in current relationships: _____

Review this assessment every few months as your relationship patterns change and your capacity for healthy connection grows.

The Heart of Healing

Relationships provide both the context where trauma often occurs and the environment where the deepest healing becomes possible. Your growing capacity for somatic awareness, self-regulation, and co-regulation creates the foundation for more authentic, satisfying connections with others.

The work you've done throughout this book—developing body awareness, learning to regulate your nervous system, and building capacity for emotional expression—all serves the ultimate goal of being able to love and be loved more fully. Your individual healing supports your relational healing, just as healthy relationships support your continued individual growth.

The final chapter explores how to integrate all these capacities into a sustainable way of living that honors your nervous system's needs while fully engaging with life's opportunities and challenges.

Relationship Healing Foundations:

- Your nervous system heals through safe connection with others as well as individual work
- Co-regulation and self-regulation both contribute to nervous system health and relationship satisfaction
- Attachment patterns can be updated through new experiences of safe, responsive connection
- Eye contact, synchronized breathing, and appropriate touch provide direct co-regulation opportunities
- Conflict can be navigated while maintaining nervous system regulation and authentic expression
- Understanding your relationship patterns helps you choose connections that support your healing
- Individual nervous system capacity directly affects your ability to maintain healthy relationships

Chapter 11: Living Somatically

Living somatically means organizing your daily life around your body's wisdom rather than overriding its messages in service of external demands or old conditioning patterns. This represents a fundamental shift from the disconnected, push-through mentality that characterizes much of modern life. When you live somatically, your nervous system becomes your primary guidance system for making decisions about work, relationships, self-care, and life direction.

This final content chapter addresses the practical challenges of maintaining your somatic awareness and regulation skills while navigating a world that often doesn't support embodied living. You'll learn to protect your gains, prevent re-traumatization, and continue growing throughout your life.

Making Somatic Awareness a Lifestyle

Transforming somatic practices from occasional interventions into a way of living requires consistent attention to how your nervous system responds to various life choices. This doesn't mean becoming self-absorbed or avoiding all challenges, but rather making decisions from an informed understanding of your capacity and needs.

Living somatically involves regular check-ins with your nervous system, environmental modifications that support your well-being, and lifestyle choices that honor your particular constitution and healing needs. This often requires changing patterns that have been automatic for years or decades.

Dr. Arielle Schwartz's research on post-traumatic growth demonstrates that trauma survivors who maintain long-term healing often develop what she calls "embodied resilience"—the ability to respond to life's challenges from a grounded, resourced place rather than reactive survival patterns (30).

Consider the case of Patricia, a 51-year-old nonprofit director who had completed several years of trauma therapy and felt significantly better. However, she noticed that her old patterns of overwhelm and anxiety would return whenever life became particularly stressful, suggesting that her healing hadn't yet become integrated into her daily lifestyle.

Patricia realized she had been treating her somatic practices as remedial interventions—things she did when she felt bad—rather than preventive lifestyle choices that maintained her well-being. Her nervous system would gradually dysregulate through accumulated stress until she reached crisis points that required intensive self-care.

Patricia began reorganizing her daily life around nervous system maintenance rather than crisis management. She started each day with a brief somatic check-in to assess her capacity and needs. She modified her work schedule to include regular breaks for nervous system regulation. She learned to say no to commitments that exceeded her current capacity.

The transformation occurred gradually as Patricia's choices became increasingly informed by her body's wisdom. She changed her commute to avoid rush hour stress, modified her office environment to include plants and natural lighting, and established boundaries around after-hours work communication.

Patricia also learned to navigate social and professional situations from an embodied place. She would track her nervous system responses during meetings and make subtle adjustments—shifting her posture, breathing consciously, or taking brief breaks—to maintain regulation throughout challenging interactions.

Most significantly, Patricia began making larger life decisions based on how they affected her nervous system. She turned down a promotion that would have required frequent travel because her body signaled that this would exceed her current capacity. She chose to relocate to a quieter neighborhood that better supported her nervous system's need for peace.

Patricia's colleagues and friends noticed that she seemed more present, authentic, and resilient. Her work performance actually improved as she learned to operate from a regulated nervous system rather than pushing through stress and overwhelm.

Preventing Re-traumatization

Once you've developed nervous system resilience and regulation skills, protecting these gains becomes essential for long-term healing. Re-traumatization can occur when you place yourself in situations that exceed your current capacity or when you revert to old patterns of overriding your nervous system's protective signals.

Prevention involves both external choices—avoiding unnecessarily traumatizing situations—and internal capacity building that increases your ability to navigate unavoidable challenges without losing your center.

The goal isn't to avoid all stress or challenge, which would limit your growth and life satisfaction. Rather, you learn to distinguish between challenges that build capacity and those that overwhelm your nervous system in ways that recreate trauma dynamics.

Consider the case of Michael, a 39-year-old teacher who had healed significantly from childhood abuse trauma. He felt confident in his recovery until he took a new job at a school where the principal's management style closely resembled his abusive father's authoritarian patterns.

Initially, Michael tried to use his regulation skills to manage his responses to the principal's behavior. However, he found himself gradually sliding back into hypervigilance, people-pleasing, and anxiety patterns that he hadn't experienced in years. His nervous system was being re-traumatized by the daily exposure to authoritarian dynamics.

Michael learned to distinguish between situations that challenged his growth edge versus those that recreated trauma dynamics. The new job wasn't just difficult—it was reactivating specific patterns of powerlessness and fear that characterized his childhood trauma.

Michael made the difficult decision to leave the job, despite external pressures to "toughen up" and "work through it." He recognized that protecting his healing was more important than meeting external expectations about resilience or persistence.

Michael found a new position in a school environment that felt collaborative and supportive rather than authoritarian. His nervous system quickly returned to its regulated baseline, confirming that the previous environment had been genuinely harmful rather than just challenging.

This experience taught Michael to trust his nervous system's feedback about environmental safety rather than pushing through activation in the name of growth or responsibility. He developed criteria for assessing whether situations were supportive challenges versus potential re-traumatization.

Michael also built stronger internal resources for navigating unavoidable difficult situations. He developed practices for maintaining his center during conflict, strategies for protecting his energy in negative environments, and skills for advocating for his needs in professional settings.

Continued Growth and Development

Somatic healing doesn't end with symptom resolution or achieving a particular level of nervous system stability. Your body and nervous system continue to have new capacities available throughout your life, and maintaining curiosity about this ongoing development prevents stagnation and supports continued vitality.

Advanced somatic development might involve increased emotional range, greater capacity for creativity and expression, enhanced intuition and decision-making, or deeper spiritual connection. These developments often emerge naturally as your nervous system becomes more regulated and integrated.

Continued growth also involves expanding your capacity to handle life's complexities without losing your center. As you heal, you may find yourself able to engage with challenges that previously would have overwhelmed you, or to contribute to others' healing in ways that weren't possible during your early recovery.

Consider the case of Sarah, a 46-year-old social worker who had spent years healing from complex trauma. She reached a point where her symptoms had largely resolved and her daily life felt manageable and satisfying. However, she began feeling restless and wondering what came after basic healing.

Sarah realized that her nervous system had developed capacity that she wasn't fully utilizing. She felt called to explore more advanced aspects of somatic development—creativity, intuition, and spiritual connection that hadn't been accessible during her survival and early healing phases.

Sarah began exploring expressive arts, meditation practices, and nature-based spirituality. She found that her nervous system could now handle states of expanded awareness and emotional intensity that would have been overwhelming earlier in her healing process.

Sarah also felt drawn to contribute to collective healing in ways that built on her personal recovery. She began facilitating support groups for trauma survivors, finding that her embodied presence and regulation skills created safety for others' healing processes.

The most surprising development was Sarah's increasing capacity for joy and spontaneity. As her nervous system released old protective patterns, she discovered aspects of herself that had been dormant for decades—playfulness, curiosity, and a capacity for delight that transformed her experience of daily life.

Sarah's continued development reminded her that healing isn't about returning to a previous state but about discovering capacities that may never have been available before. Her trauma recovery had opened possibilities for growth that exceeded her pre-trauma functioning.

Exercise 11.1: Daily Life Movement Practices

Integrating movement into your daily activities helps maintain nervous system regulation without requiring separate time for formal exercise. These practices help you stay embodied and present throughout your day while supporting your nervous system's need for movement and circulation.

The goal is developing a repertoire of simple movements that can be done anywhere, anytime you notice tension, stagnation, or disconnection from your body.

Morning Activation Sequence Begin each day with simple movements that help your nervous system transition from sleep to active engagement:

Gentle Stretching: While still in bed, stretch your arms overhead, point and flex your feet, and gently twist your spine to awaken your body.

Joint Mobility: Slowly move each joint through its range of motion—ankles, knees, hips, shoulders, and neck—to promote circulation and flexibility.

Spinal Wave: Stand and create gentle wave-like movements through your spine, starting from your pelvis and moving up through your neck.

Energy Activation: Use gentle bouncing, arm swinging, or marching in place to activate your circulation and nervous system for the day ahead.

Workplace Movement Integration Incorporate nervous system supporting movements into your work environment:

Hourly Movement Breaks: Set reminders to move for 1-2 minutes every hour—standing, stretching, walking, or doing simple exercises at your desk.

Micro-Movement: Practice subtle movements throughout your workday—toe wiggles, shoulder rolls, neck stretches, or breathing exercises that don't disrupt your work.

Posture Resets: Regularly check and adjust your posture, feeling your feet on the ground, lengthening your spine, and releasing unnecessary tension.

Stress Discharge: When you notice stress accumulation, use brief movement to discharge activation—hand shaking, shoulder shrugging, or gentle self-massage.

Transition Movement Rituals Create movement practices that help you transition between different activities or environments:

Leaving Work: Develop a brief movement sequence that helps you transition from work mode to personal time—stretching, walking, or breathing exercises.

Entering Home: Create a ritual of movement that helps you arrive fully in your home space—hanging up work clothes mindfully, washing hands with awareness, or briefly moving your body.

Before Meals: Use simple movements to help your nervous system shift into rest-and-digest mode—gentle stretching, deep breathing, or brief walking.

Evening Wind-Down: Develop calming movements that prepare your nervous system for sleep—gentle yoga, stretching, or slow, flowing movements.

Social Movement Integration Practice embodied awareness during social interactions:

Walking Meetings: When appropriate, conduct meetings or conversations while walking, which can support nervous system regulation for both people.

Embodied Listening: Practice staying connected to your body while listening to others, noticing your physical responses to different types of conversation.

Social Boundary Awareness: Use subtle movement to maintain your energetic boundaries during social interactions—feeling your feet, adjusting posture, or using breathing to stay centered.

Group Regulation: In group settings, use your embodied presence to contribute to collective nervous system regulation through your own groundedness and calm.

Exercise 11.2: Workplace Regulation Techniques

Work environments often challenge your nervous system through stress, conflict, deadlines, and social dynamics. Developing regulation techniques that work in professional settings helps you maintain your well-being while meeting work responsibilities.

These techniques should be subtle enough to use without drawing unwanted attention while effective enough to maintain your nervous system regulation throughout challenging workdays.

Discrete Breathing Techniques Practice breathing exercises that can be done during meetings, phone calls, or while working at your computer:

Silent Coherent Breathing: Practice 5-5 breathing (5 seconds in, 5 seconds out) silently while participating in meetings or conversations.

Physiological Sighs: Use the double inhale, long exhale pattern discretely when you notice stress accumulation.

Belly Breathing: Place one hand on your belly under your desk and practice deep breathing that activates your parasympathetic nervous system.

Breath Awareness: Simply maintaining awareness of your breath throughout the day provides ongoing nervous system support without requiring specific techniques.

Grounding and Presence Practices Stay connected to your body and present moment awareness during work activities:

Feet on Floor: Regularly feel your feet on the ground, using this connection to maintain embodied presence during stressful situations.

Body Check-Ins: Periodically scan your body for tension or holding patterns, making small adjustments to maintain comfort and openness.

Sensory Awareness: Practice 5-4-3-2-1 grounding (5 things you see, 4 you feel, 3 you hear, 2 you smell, 1 you taste) during overwhelming moments.

Present Moment Anchoring: Use your breath, body position, or environmental awareness to stay present during anxiety-provoking situations.

Stress Discharge Techniques Develop ways to discharge stress accumulation throughout your workday:

Bathroom Breaks: Use restroom visits as opportunities for brief stress discharge through movement, stretching, or conscious breathing.

Stairwell Movement: If possible, use stairs as opportunities for physical movement that helps discharge nervous system activation.

Hand and Arm Exercises: Practice discrete hand clenching and releasing, arm stretching, or shoulder rolling while sitting at your desk.

Vocal Discharge: Use private moments (in your car, office with door closed) for brief vocal stress release through sighing, humming, or quiet toning.

Interpersonal Regulation Strategies Maintain your nervous system regulation during challenging interpersonal interactions at work:

Boundary Awareness: Practice maintaining your energetic boundaries during meetings or conflicts through posture, breathing, and internal awareness.

Conflict Regulation: Use breathing and grounding techniques to stay present and regulated during workplace conflicts or difficult conversations.

Co-Regulation Opportunities: When appropriate, use your regulated presence to contribute to calmer group dynamics during stressful meetings or deadlines.

Recovery Practices: Develop routines for recovering from particularly challenging interpersonal interactions—brief walks, breathing exercises, or calling supportive friends.

Environmental Modifications Make changes to your work environment that support nervous system regulation:

Lighting Adjustments: Use natural light when possible, adjust computer screen brightness, or add lamps that create more comfortable lighting.

Sound Management: Use headphones, white noise, or nature sounds to create more supportive auditory environments when possible.

Personal Items: Include plants, photos, or other items that provide nervous system resources and remind you of safety and support.

Ergonomic Awareness: Adjust your workspace to support comfortable posture and reduce physical stress that contributes to nervous system dysregulation.

Exercise 11.3: Somatic Parenting Basics

Parenting from an embodied place helps you respond to your children's needs while maintaining your own nervous system regulation. This approach benefits both you and your children by modeling healthy self-care and providing the calm, attuned presence that children need for optimal development.

Somatic parenting involves using your body's wisdom to guide your responses to parenting challenges while teaching your children basic emotional regulation and body awareness skills.

Nervous System Co-Regulation with Children Use your regulated nervous system to help your children develop their own regulation capacity:

Calm Presence: When your child is upset, focus first on regulating your own nervous system before trying to help them. Children co-regulate with their parents' nervous system state.

Breathing Together: Teach children simple breathing exercises and practice them together during calm moments and stressful situations.

Physical Comfort: Use appropriate touch—hand on back, holding, or hugging—to provide nervous system co-regulation when children are distressed.

Emotional Attunement: Reflect your child's emotional state while remaining grounded in your own regulation: "You seem really frustrated right now, and that makes sense."

Teaching Body Awareness to Children Help children develop their own somatic awareness and regulation skills:

Feeling Check-Ins: Regularly ask children how their bodies feel, helping them develop vocabulary for physical sensations and emotions.

Movement Integration: Encourage regular movement, dancing, or active play that supports children's nervous system regulation and development.

Breathing Games: Teach children breathing techniques through play—blowing bubbles, pretending to be sleeping bears, or practicing "flower and candle" breathing.

Body Boundary Education: Teach children about personal space, appropriate touch, and their right to say no to unwanted physical contact.

Parental Self-Care and Regulation Maintain your own nervous system health while meeting parenting demands:

Regular Self-Assessment: Check in with your nervous system throughout the day, noticing when you need breaks or support.

Micro-Recovery Practices: Use brief moments for nervous system regulation—conscious breathing while children play, stretching during quiet time, or grounding exercises.

Parenting Triggers: Develop awareness of situations that trigger your own childhood trauma or overwhelm, creating strategies for staying regulated during these challenges.

Support Networks: Build relationships with other parents who understand the importance of nervous system health in parenting.

Responding to Children's Emotions Use somatic awareness to respond appropriately to children's emotional expressions:

Tantrum Regulation: Stay grounded and present during children's emotional outbursts, providing calm witnessing rather than trying to immediately stop the expression.

Emotional Validation: Acknowledge children's emotions while maintaining your own boundaries: "I can see you're angry, and hitting isn't okay."

Teaching Emotional Expression: Help children learn healthy ways to express difficult emotions through movement, art, or appropriate vocal expression.

Modeling Regulation: Demonstrate healthy emotional expression and regulation in your own responses to stress and challenge.

Family Nervous System Awareness Create family practices that support everyone's nervous system health:

Family Movement Time: Establish regular times for family dance, walks, or active play that supports everyone's nervous system regulation.

Calm Spaces: Create areas in your home designed for quiet, regulation, and restoration that all family members can use.

Routine and Predictability: Maintain predictable routines that support children's nervous system development while remaining flexible when needed.

Conflict Resolution: Teach family members to take breaks during conflicts when nervous systems become activated, returning to problem-solving from regulated states.

Exercise 11.4: Community and Collective Healing

Your individual healing contributes to collective healing, and engaging with community healing efforts can support your continued growth while serving the larger world. This exercise explores ways to extend your somatic awareness into community engagement and social contribution.

Collective healing recognizes that individual trauma often has social and cultural roots, and that creating healthier communities supports everyone's nervous system health and resilience.

Community Nervous System Awareness Develop sensitivity to the nervous system health of groups and communities you participate in:

Group Energy Assessment: Notice how your nervous system responds to different groups—family gatherings, work meetings, social organizations, or spiritual communities.

Collective Activation Patterns: Observe how stress, excitement, conflict, or joy moves through groups and affects individual nervous systems.

Community Resources: Identify communities that support your nervous system health and consider how you might contribute to their collective well-being.

Social Nervous System Impact: Notice how larger social events—elections, disasters, celebrations—affect your and others' nervous system functioning.

Contributing to Collective Regulation Use your regulated presence to support community nervous system health:

Modeling Regulation: Bring your embodied presence to group situations, contributing to collective calm through your own groundedness.

Conflict Mediation: Use your nervous system awareness to help de-escalate group conflicts or facilitate difficult conversations.

Teaching and Sharing: Share somatic awareness skills with others through formal or informal teaching, modeling, or mentoring.

Creating Safe Spaces: Help organize or facilitate groups that prioritize nervous system safety and emotional regulation.

Addressing Collective Trauma Engage with healing work that addresses community and cultural trauma patterns:

Historical Trauma Awareness: Learn about historical trauma that affects your community or cultural group, understanding how past events influence current nervous system patterns.

Social Justice Engagement: Participate in efforts to address systemic issues that create ongoing trauma for marginalized communities.

Community Healing Circles: Join or organize groups focused on collective processing and healing of shared traumatic experiences.

Cultural Reclamation: Engage with practices that help restore cultural traditions or ways of being that support nervous system health.

Environmental and Ecological Healing Recognize the connection between environmental health and nervous system well-being:

Nature Connection: Spend regular time in natural environments that support nervous system regulation and remember your connection to larger ecological systems.

Environmental Advocacy: Engage in protecting natural spaces and addressing environmental issues that affect community health and well-being.

Sustainable Living: Make lifestyle choices that reflect your understanding of the interconnection between personal and planetary health.

Ecological Nervous System: Develop awareness of how environmental destruction and restoration affect collective nervous system health.

Building Healing Communities Create or participate in communities that actively support nervous system health and trauma healing:

Mutual Support Networks: Develop relationships with others committed to healing and growth who can provide ongoing support and accountability.

Healing-Centered Organizations: Participate in or create organizations that prioritize trauma-informed practices and nervous system awareness.

Intergenerational Healing: Engage in efforts to break cycles of trauma transmission and support healing across age groups.

Resource Sharing: Share knowledge, skills, and resources that support collective healing and nervous system health.

Final Assessment: Progress Celebration

Take time to acknowledge the journey you've traveled and the capacities you've developed through this somatic healing work. This assessment helps you recognize your growth while identifying areas for continued development.

Nervous System Capacity Assessment Compare your current nervous system functioning to when you began this work:

Regulation Skills: How has your ability to self-regulate improved? What techniques have become most reliable for you?

Window of Tolerance: Has your capacity to handle stress and activation expanded? Do you notice greater flexibility in your responses?

Body Awareness: How has your relationship with your body changed? What do you notice now that you couldn't sense before?

Emotional Range: Has your capacity to feel and express emotions expanded? Which emotions feel more accessible now?

Relationship Capacity: How have your relationships changed as your nervous system has healed? What new capacities do you have for connection?

Healing Integration Assessment Evaluate how well you've integrated somatic practices into your daily life:

Daily Practice: Which practices have become natural parts of your routine? What feels sustainable for long-term maintenance?

Challenge Navigation: How do you handle stress and difficulties differently than before? What resources do you reach for during challenging times?

Decision Making: How has your decision-making process changed? Do you include your body's wisdom in important choices?

Lifestyle Alignment: What changes have you made to align your life more closely with your nervous system needs?

Continued Growth Planning: What areas of somatic development feel most important for your next phase of growth?

Appreciation and Acknowledgment Take time to fully appreciate the courage and commitment you've shown in this healing work:

Personal Courage: Acknowledge the bravery it takes to face trauma and develop new ways of being in your body.

Consistency and Commitment: Appreciate your willingness to practice consistently even when progress felt slow or invisible.

Vulnerability and Openness: Honor your willingness to be vulnerable in service of healing and growth.

Community Support: Acknowledge the people who have supported your healing journey and express gratitude for their presence.

Future Vision: Set intentions for how you want to continue living somatically and contributing to collective healing.

Worksheet: Future Vision and Goals

Creating a clear vision for your continued somatic development helps maintain momentum while providing direction for your ongoing growth and healing.

Long-Term Somatic Vision Imagine your life five years from now, living fully from somatic awareness:

How do you want to feel in your body on a daily basis? _____ What capacity for stress and challenge do you want to have? _____ How do you want your relationships to feel and function? _____ What contribution do you want to make to collective healing? _____ What aspects of yourself do you want to continue developing? _____

One-Year Somatic Goals Set specific, achievable goals for the next year:

Nervous System Development: What regulation capacity do you want to build over the next year? _____

Body Relationship: How do you want your relationship with your body to deepen? _____

Emotional Capacity: What emotional development feels most important for you? _____

Relationship Growth: How do you want your relationship capacity to expand? _____

Life Integration: What lifestyle changes do you want to make to support your nervous system? _____

Quarterly Milestone Planning Break down your yearly goals into quarterly milestones:

Quarter 1 Focus: What specific practices or developments do you want to focus on in the next three months? _____

Quarter 2 Goals: What capacity do you want to build in months 4-6? _____

Quarter 3 Expansion: How do you want to expand or deepen your practice in months 7-9? _____

Quarter 4 Integration: What integration or lifestyle changes do you want to complete by year's end? _____

Monthly Practice Planning Create sustainable monthly practice goals:

Daily Practice Commitment: What daily somatic practices feel sustainable and nourishing? _____

Weekly Expansion: What weekly practices or challenges do you want to include? _____

Monthly Assessment: How will you track your progress and adjust your practices? _____

Seasonal Adaptations: How will you modify your practices based on seasonal changes and life circumstances? _____

Support and Accountability Planning Identify support for your continued development:

Professional Support: What ongoing professional support do you need (therapy, bodywork, training)? _____

Community Connection: What communities or groups will support your continued growth? _____

Peer Accountability: Who can provide ongoing support and accountability for your practice? _____

Learning and Development: What additional training or education will support your growth? _____

Resource Planning: What books, apps, or other resources will support your continued development? _____

Obstacle Preparation Plan for challenges that might interfere with your continued growth:

Life Stress Management: How will you maintain your practices during particularly stressful periods? _____

Motivation Fluctuations: What will you do during times when motivation feels low? _____

Relapse Prevention: How will you handle temporary returns to old patterns without giving up? _____

Support During Challenges: Who can you reach out to when facing particular difficulties? _____

Practice Adaptation: How will you modify your practices for illness, travel, or major life changes? _____

Contribution and Service Goals Plan how your healing will serve others and contribute to collective healing:

Sharing Your Growth: How do you want to share what you've learned with others? _____

Community Contribution: What communities do you want to contribute to through your somatic awareness?

_____

Professional Integration: How might you integrate somatic awareness into your work or career? _____

Family and Relationship Impact: How will your continued growth serve your family and close relationships?

_____

Social Healing Participation: How do you want to participate in larger social healing efforts? _____

Your Somatic Life Awaits

Living somatically represents a return to your body's innate wisdom while integrating the skills and capacities you've developed through conscious healing work. This isn't a destination but an ongoing journey of deepening relationship with yourself and the world around you.

Your nervous system's capacity for growth and adaptation continues throughout your life. The practices and awareness you've developed through this workbook provide a foundation for continued development that can support not only your individual well-being but also your contribution to collective healing and social transformation.

As you continue this journey, trust your body's wisdom to guide you toward the experiences, relationships, and contributions that will support your continued growth. Your healing serves not only yourself but also the larger web of connection of which you are a part.

The path of somatic healing leads ultimately to a life of greater authenticity, resilience, and capacity for both giving and receiving love. Your willingness to undertake this journey represents not only personal courage but also a contribution to the healing of our collective trauma and the creation of a more embodied, compassionate world.

Living Somatically - Essential Principles:

- Somatic awareness becomes a lifestyle through consistent attention to your nervous system's needs and responses
- Preventing re-traumatization requires distinguishing between growth challenges and harmful situations
- Continued development includes expanding emotional range, creativity, and capacity for contribution
- Daily movement practices maintain nervous system regulation without requiring separate exercise time
- Workplace regulation techniques help you maintain well-being in professional environments

- Somatic parenting models nervous system health while supporting children's development
- Community engagement extends individual healing into collective transformation
- Your continued growth serves both personal fulfillment and social healing

Chapter 12: Your Ongoing Journey - Resources and Next Steps

The work you've accomplished through this workbook represents the beginning rather than the end of your somatic healing journey. Your growing nervous system capacity, body awareness, and regulation skills create a foundation for continued development that can unfold throughout your lifetime. This final chapter provides practical guidance for maintaining your progress while expanding your knowledge and skills through additional resources and support.

Your healing journey is unique, and the next steps that serve you best will depend on your individual circumstances, interests, and goals. Some people feel ready to deepen their practice through additional training or therapy, while others focus on integrating what they've learned into their daily lives. Trust your body's wisdom to guide you toward the resources and opportunities that will best support your continued growth.

When and How to Find a Somatic Therapist

Professional somatic therapy can provide support that goes beyond what self-directed practice can accomplish. Working with a skilled somatic therapist offers the benefit of external nervous system regulation, professional guidance through challenging territory, and specialized interventions for complex trauma patterns.

The decision to seek professional support often arises when you encounter patterns that feel stuck despite consistent self-practice, when you want to deepen your healing beyond what feels possible alone, or when life circumstances create challenges that exceed your current coping capacity.

Dr. Susan Aposhyan's research indicates that the therapeutic relationship itself provides a crucial healing environment for nervous system regulation and attachment repair (31). The safety and attunement of a skilled therapist can help you access and integrate experiences that might be too overwhelming to approach alone.

Consider the timing carefully. Some people benefit from professional support at the beginning of their healing journey to establish safety and basic regulation skills. Others develop these capacities through self-practice before adding professional support for deeper work. Still others integrate periods of therapy with independent practice throughout their healing journey.

Identifying Your Readiness for Professional Support You might benefit from professional somatic therapy if you experience:

- Trauma responses that feel too overwhelming to work with alone
- Patterns that remain stuck despite consistent self-practice
- Dissociation that interferes with daily functioning
- Relationship difficulties that stem from nervous system dysregulation
- Complex trauma that requires specialized intervention
- A desire to deepen your understanding and capacity beyond self-directed work

Finding Qualified Somatic Therapists Look for practitioners who have completed training in established somatic modalities such as:

- Somatic Experience (SE) developed by Peter Levine
- Hakomi Method created by Ron Kurtz
- Sensorimotor Psychotherapy founded by Pat Ogden
- NARM (NeuroAffective Relational Model) developed by Laurence Heller

- Body-Mind Psychotherapy or other recognized somatic approaches

Verify credentials through the training organizations' websites, which typically maintain directories of certified practitioners. Look for therapists who have completed at least basic certification in their chosen modality, with additional preference for those who have pursued advanced training.

Evaluating Therapeutic Fit The relationship between you and your therapist matters as much as their technical qualifications. During initial consultations, assess:

- How your nervous system responds to the therapist's presence
- Their understanding of trauma and nervous system functioning
- Their approach to pacing and respecting your capacity
- Their ability to explain their methods clearly
- Your sense of feeling seen and understood by them

Trust your somatic responses during initial meetings. If you feel activated, judged, or misunderstood, continue looking. The right therapeutic relationship should feel supportive and regulation-promoting from the beginning.

Working Effectively with Somatic Therapists Maximize your therapeutic experience by:

- Communicating openly about your nervous system responses during sessions
- Practicing techniques between sessions and reporting your experiences
- Being honest about what feels helpful versus unhelpful
- Asking questions about the therapeutic process and rationale

- Maintaining your own self-care practices alongside therapy

Remember that you are the expert on your own experience. A skilled somatic therapist will welcome your feedback and collaborate with you in designing interventions that serve your unique needs.

Recommended Training Programs

Formal training in somatic modalities can deepen your understanding while potentially preparing you to support others' healing. Training programs range from introductory workshops for personal development to professional certification programs for therapists and healers.

Many people find that learning about nervous system functioning and somatic interventions enhances their own healing even if they don't intend to work professionally in the field. Understanding the theory behind the practices often increases their effectiveness and helps you apply them more skillfully.

Professional Training Programs If you're interested in becoming a somatic practitioner, research programs carefully:

Somatic Experiencing (SE): Three-year training program leading to practitioner certification. Focuses on nervous system regulation and trauma resolution through titrated exposure and discharge.

Hakomi Method: Multi-year training emphasizing mindfulness, non-violence, and holism. Integrates body awareness, movement, and verbal processing.

Sensorimotor Psychotherapy: Training for licensed therapists to integrate body-based interventions into their practice. Emphasizes movement, posture, and nervous system regulation.

NeuroAffective Relational Model (NARM): Focuses on developmental trauma and attachment repair through nervous system regulation and relational healing.

Somatic Transformation Institute: Offers various programs integrating multiple somatic approaches with emphasis on social justice and community healing.

Each program has different requirements, time commitments, and costs. Most require previous experience in healthcare, mental health, or related fields. Research prerequisites carefully before applying.

Personal Development Training For those interested in deepening personal practice rather than professional work:

Introductory Workshops: Most training organizations offer weekend workshops or short courses for personal development. These provide valuable learning without major time or financial commitments.

Online Learning: Many organizations now offer online courses, making training more accessible to people in remote areas or with scheduling constraints.

Retreat Programs: Intensive retreat experiences can provide deep personal work while learning somatic principles and practices.

Community Education: Look for community centers, yoga studios, or wellness centers that offer somatic-based classes or workshops.

Continuing Education for Professionals If you're already a healthcare or mental health professional:

Many somatic training programs offer continuing education credits for licensed professionals. This allows you to integrate somatic approaches into your existing practice while meeting professional development requirements.

Research whether training programs are approved for continuing education in your profession and state. Requirements vary significantly across different licensing boards.

Building Your Support Network

Healing happens in community as much as in individual practice. Building a network of people who understand and support your somatic healing journey provides ongoing resources for growth, accountability for your practices, and community for sharing your experiences.

Your support network might include family members and friends who respect your healing process, fellow travelers on similar journeys, professional supporters like therapists or bodyworkers, and communities organized around somatic principles or trauma healing.

Family and Friend Support Help the important people in your life understand your healing journey:

- Share information about nervous system functioning and somatic healing when appropriate
- Communicate your needs clearly rather than expecting others to intuitively understand
- Set boundaries around discussions or behaviors that interfere with your healing
- Appreciate support while maintaining responsibility for your own healing process

- Model the nervous system regulation and embodied presence you're developing

Not everyone in your life will understand or support your healing journey. Focus your energy on relationships that feel nourishing while maintaining appropriate boundaries with those who don't.

Peer Support Communities Connect with others who share similar healing goals:

- Online communities focused on trauma healing or somatic practices
- Local support groups for trauma survivors or people interested in embodied living
- Workshops or classes where you can meet like-minded people
- Social media groups dedicated to nervous system health and somatic awareness
- Informal networks that develop around shared interests in healing and growth

Choose communities that feel supportive rather than competitive or triggering. Healthy healing communities encourage individual growth while providing mutual support and understanding.

Professional Support Team Consider assembling a team of professionals who support different aspects of your healing:

- Primary healthcare provider who understands trauma and nervous system health
- Mental health therapist trained in somatic or trauma-informed approaches
- Bodyworker (massage therapist, acupuncturist, chiropractor) who understands trauma
- Movement professional (yoga teacher, dance therapist, personal trainer) with somatic training

- Spiritual advisor or mentor who honors embodied spirituality

You don't need all these professionals, but having a few trusted practitioners who understand your healing approach can provide valuable support during challenging periods.

Continuing Education Options

Your understanding of nervous system functioning, trauma recovery, and somatic healing can continue developing throughout your life. Staying current with new research and developments in the field keeps your practice fresh while expanding your capacity for growth and healing.

The field of somatic healing continues evolving rapidly, with new research, techniques, and applications emerging regularly. Ongoing education helps you benefit from these developments while deepening your existing knowledge and skills.

Books and Written Resources Continue expanding your knowledge through reading:

Foundational Texts:

- "Waking the Tiger" by Peter Levine
- "The Body Keeps the Score" by Bessel van der Kolk
- "Trauma and the Body" by Pat Ogden
- "The Mindful Body" by Ellen Langer
- "Full Catastrophe Living" by Jon Kabat-Zinn

Advanced Reading:

- "In an Unspoken Voice" by Peter Levine
- "The NeuroAffective Relational Model" by Laurence Heller

- "The Pocket Guide to the Polyvagal Theory" by Stephen Porges
- "Healing Trauma" by Peter Levine
- "The Revolution Will Not Be Therapized" by Sara David

Online Learning Platforms Many organizations offer online courses and webinars:

- Somatic Experiencing International provides regular webinars and online training
- The Embodiment Institute offers various online programs
- Sounds True features numerous somatic and trauma healing courses
- Learning and Development Center provides trauma-informed training
- YouTube channels of reputable somatic practitioners offer free educational content

Conferences and Workshops Attend events that focus on somatic healing and nervous system health:

- International conferences on trauma and healing
- Regional workshops offered by training organizations
- Local wellness centers or yoga studios hosting somatic practitioners
- Online summits and virtual conferences
- University continuing education programs

Research and Scientific Literature For those interested in the scientific foundations:

- Journal of Traumatic Stress
- Clinical Psychology Review
- Frontiers in Psychology
- Applied Psychology: Health and Well-Being

- Google Scholar alerts for "somatic therapy," "nervous system regulation," "trauma recovery"

Stay curious while maintaining discernment. Not all new approaches or research will be relevant to your particular healing journey.

Creating Healing Communities

Your individual healing naturally extends into creating communities that support collective nervous system health and trauma recovery. This might involve formal organization of support groups or healing circles, or simply modeling embodied presence in your existing communities.

Creating healing communities serves both your continued growth and your contribution to collective healing. When you help create spaces where others can experience nervous system safety and regulation, you also benefit from the co-regulating effects of being in such environments.

Starting Support Groups Consider organizing groups focused on somatic healing and nervous system health:

Peer Support Groups: Gather people interested in practicing somatic techniques together. These groups can provide accountability, shared learning, and mutual support without requiring professional leadership.

Practice Groups: Organize regular meetings focused on practicing specific techniques like breathing exercises, movement practices, or meditation. Having others to practice with can maintain motivation and provide shared learning.

Study Groups: Form groups to read and discuss books about nervous system health, trauma recovery, or somatic healing.

Combining intellectual understanding with embodied practice often deepens learning.

Community Healing Circles: Create opportunities for people to share their healing journeys while practicing supportive listening and nervous system regulation together.

Contributing to Existing Communities Bring somatic awareness to communities you already participate in:

Workplace Wellness: Share stress management and nervous system regulation techniques in your workplace. Offer to lead brief relaxation sessions or teach breathing exercises.

Family Integration: Model embodied presence in your family relationships. Teach children basic body awareness and emotional regulation skills appropriate for their development.

Spiritual Communities: Integrate somatic awareness into your spiritual practice or religious community. Many traditions welcome body-based approaches to spiritual development.

Social Justice Work: Apply nervous system awareness to activism and social justice efforts. Help create sustainable approaches to social change that don't re-traumatize participants.

Online Community Building Use technology to create virtual healing communities:

- Start social media groups focused on somatic healing and nervous system health
- Create online practice partners or accountability groups
- Share educational content that helps others learn about embodied healing
- Participate constructively in existing online communities
- Use video conferencing for virtual practice groups or support meetings

Maintain the same principles online that you would use in person—prioritizing safety, consent, and nervous system regulation in all interactions.

Professional Directory Guide

Finding qualified practitioners can be challenging, especially in areas with limited somatic therapy resources. This directory guide provides starting points for locating trained professionals while emphasizing the importance of personal fit over credentials alone.

Major Training Organization Directories Most somatic training organizations maintain directories of certified practitioners:

Somatic Experiencing International Website: traumahealing.org Provides searchable directory of SE practitioners worldwide Includes practitioner contact information and training levels

Hakomi Institute
Website: hakomiinstitute.com Directory of certified Hakomi practitioners and therapists Includes information about practitioner specialties and approaches

Sensorimotor Psychotherapy Institute Website: sensorimotorpsychotherapy.org Directory limited to licensed mental health professionals trained in SP Includes location and contact information for certified therapists

NARM Institute Website: theartofinnerconnection.com Directory of NARM practitioners and training candidates Focuses on developmental trauma and attachment repair

Professional Association Directories Mental health and bodywork associations often include somatic practitioners:

International Association of Marriage and Family Counselors Many IAMFC members have training in somatic approaches to couples and family therapy

American Massage Therapy Association Some AMTA members specialize in trauma-informed massage and bodywork

International Association of Yoga Therapists IAYT members often integrate somatic awareness into yoga-based healing

Psychology Today Directory Many somatic therapists list their services and specialties on this widely-used platform

Evaluation Criteria for Practitioners When researching potential therapists or practitioners, consider:

Training Background: What formal training have they completed? Are they certified by recognized training organizations?

Professional Licensing: Do they hold appropriate professional licenses for their scope of practice?

Experience Level: How long have they been practicing? Do they have experience with your particular concerns?

Approach and Philosophy: Do their described approaches align with your healing goals and values?

Accessibility: Are their location, scheduling, and fees workable for your situation?

Referral Network: Can they provide referrals to other practitioners if needed?

Questions for Initial Consultations During preliminary conversations with potential practitioners, ask:

- What is your training background in somatic approaches?
- How do you typically work with nervous system regulation?
- What experience do you have with my particular concerns?
- How do you pace therapy to respect clients' capacity?
- What do you see as your role versus my role in the healing process?
- How do you handle situations where clients become overwhelmed?
- What additional resources or practitioners do you recommend?

Trust your nervous system responses during these conversations as much as the practitioner's verbal responses.

Alternative Practitioner Options If formally trained somatic therapists aren't available in your area, consider:

Trauma-Informed Therapists: Licensed mental health professionals with training in trauma treatment, even if not specifically somatic-trained

Bodyworkers with Trauma Training: Massage therapists, acupuncturists, or other bodyworkers who have pursued additional training in trauma-informed care

Movement Therapists: Dance/movement therapists, yoga therapists, or other movement professionals with somatic training

Spiritual Directors or Counselors: Religious or spiritual advisors who integrate body-based approaches into their practice

Online Therapy Options: Teletherapy with qualified somatic practitioners who may not be geographically accessible otherwise

Remember that the quality of the therapeutic relationship often matters more than the specific credentials or training background of the practitioner.

Your Continued Journey

The path of somatic healing extends far beyond symptom relief or trauma recovery. It opens into a way of living that honors your body's wisdom, supports your nervous system's natural capacity for resilience, and enables you to contribute to the healing of our collective trauma.

Your willingness to undertake this healing journey represents not only personal courage but also a contribution to the evolution of human consciousness toward greater embodiment, compassion, and wisdom. Each person who develops nervous system regulation and embodied presence makes it easier for others to access these capacities.

The resources and support you develop serve not only your individual healing but also your ability to create ripples of healing in your family, community, and larger world. Your embodied presence becomes a gift that you offer simply by being who you are becoming.

Trust your body's wisdom to guide you toward the next steps that will best serve your continued growth. Your nervous system knows what it needs to heal and thrive—the practices and awareness you've developed help you listen more clearly to this internal guidance.

The journey continues not because healing is never complete, but because growth and development remain possible throughout your lifetime. Your capacity for joy, creativity, connection, and contribution can continue expanding as your nervous system becomes increasingly regulated and integrated.

Resources for Continued Learning

Essential Books for Deeper Study:

- "Waking the Tiger" by Peter Levine - foundational understanding of trauma and nervous system healing
- "The Body Keeps the Score" by Bessel van der Kolk - comprehensive overview of trauma's effects and healing approaches
- "Trauma and the Body" by Pat Ogden - detailed exploration of somatic psychotherapy techniques
- "The NeuroAffective Relational Model" by Laurence Heller - focus on developmental trauma and attachment healing
- "Full Catastrophe Living" by Jon Kabat-Zinn - mindfulness-based stress reduction and embodied awareness

Training Organizations and Websites:

- Somatic Experiencing International (traumahealing.org) - largest international SE training organization
- Hakomi Institute (hakomiinstitute.com) - mindful somatic therapy training
- Sensorimotor Psychotherapy Institute (sensorimotorpsychotherapy.org) - body-oriented therapy for trauma
- NARM Institute (theartofinnerconnection.com) - developmental trauma healing approach
- The Embodiment Institute - online somatic training and resources

Professional Support Resources:

- Psychology Today directory for finding somatic therapists
- International Expressive Arts Therapy Association for creative approaches
- American Massage Therapy Association for trauma-informed bodywork
- Yoga Alliance for trauma-sensitive yoga practitioners
- Local community mental health centers for accessible trauma therapy

Online Learning and Support:

- Sounds True online courses in somatic healing and trauma recovery
- The Trauma Recovery Network for educational resources and community
- YouTube channels of established somatic practitioners
- Podcasts focused on nervous system health and embodied healing
- Virtual support groups and online practice communities

Your healing journey is both deeply personal and inherently connected to the larger web of life. As you continue growing in embodied awareness and nervous system resilience, you contribute to the collective healing that our world desperately needs. Trust the wisdom of your body to guide you toward whatever comes next in this extraordinary journey of becoming fully alive.

Essential Next Steps:

- Professional somatic therapy provides specialized support beyond self-directed practice
- Training programs offer deeper understanding whether for personal growth or professional development
- Support networks including family, peers, and professionals sustain long-term healing

- Continuing education keeps your practice current with new developments in the field
- Creating healing communities extends individual recovery into collective transformation
- Professional directories help locate qualified practitioners while emphasizing relationship fit
- Your continued journey serves both personal fulfillment and contribution to collective healing

References

(1) Levine, P. A. (2010). *In an Unspoken Voice: How the Body Releases Trauma and Restores Goodness*. North Atlantic Books.

(2) van der Kolk, B. A. (2014). *The Body Keeps the Score: Brain, Mind, and Body in the Healing of Trauma*. Viking.

(3) Damasio, A. (2018). *The Strange Order of Things: Life, Feeling, and the Making of Cultures*. Pantheon Books.

(4) Mayer, E. A. (2016). The gut-brain connection: How the hidden conversation within our bodies impacts our mood, our choices, and our overall health. *Gastroenterology*, 151(4), 733-746.

(5) Ogden, P., Minton, K., & Pain, C. (2006). *Trauma and the Body: A Sensorimotor Approach to Psychotherapy*. W. W. Norton & Company.

(6) van der Kolk, B. A. (2006). Clinical implications of neuroscience research in PTSD. *Annals of the New York Academy of Sciences*, 1071(1), 277-293.

(7) Levine, P. A. (1997). *Waking the Tiger: Healing Trauma*. North Atlantic Books.

(8) Siegel, D. J. (2012). *The Developing Mind: How Relationships and the Brain Interact to Shape Who We Are*. Guilford Press.

(9) Porges, S. W. (2011). *The Polyvagal Theory: Neurophysiological Foundations of Emotions, Attachment, Communication, and Self-Regulation*. W. W. Norton & Company.

(10) Barrett, L. F. (2017). *How Emotions Are Made: The Secret Life of the Brain*. Houghton Mifflin Harcourt.

(11) Ogden, P., & Fisher, J. (2015). *Sensorimotor Psychotherapy: Interventions for Trauma and Attachment*. W. W. Norton & Company.

(12) Porges, S. W. (2022). *Polyvagal Safety: Attachment, Communication, Self-Regulation*. W. W. Norton & Company.

(13) Brown, R. P., & Gerbarg, P. L. (2012). The healing power of the breath: Simple techniques to reduce stress and anxiety, enhance concentration, and balance your emotions. *Current Psychiatry Reports*, 14(4), 448-455.

(14) Jerath, R., Edry, J. W., Barnes, V. A., & Jerath, V. (2006). Physiology of long pranayamic breathing: Neural respiratory elements may provide a mechanism that explains how slow deep breathing shifts the autonomic nervous system. *Medical Hypotheses*, 67(3), 566-571.

(15) Epel, E., Daubenmier, J., Moskowitz, J. T., Folkman, S., & Blackburn, E. (2009). Can meditation slow rate of cellular aging? Cognitive stress, mindfulness, and telomeres. *Annals of the New York Academy of Sciences*, 1172(1), 34-53.

(16) Huberman, A. D. (2021). Controlling stress in real time. *Huberman Lab Podcast*. Stanford School of Medicine.

(17) Bercier, M. L., & Maynard, B. R. (2015). Interventions for secondary traumatic stress with mental health workers: A systematic review. *Research on Social Work Practice*, 25(1), 81-89.

(18) Bercier, M. L. (2013). Interventions that help the helpers: A systematic review and meta-analysis of interventions targeting

secondary trauma in child welfare workers. *Trauma, Violence, & Abuse*, 14(4), 334-344.

(19) Field, T. (2014). Touch for socioemotional and physical well-being: A review. *Developmental Review*, 34(2), 130-151.

(20) Field, T. (2016). Massage therapy research review. *Complementary Therapies in Clinical Practice*, 24, 19-31.

(21) Levine, P. A. (2008). *Healing Trauma: A Pioneering Program for Restoring the Wisdom of Your Body*. Sounds True.

(22) Ogden, P. (2021). The neurobiological effects of childhood trauma and the importance of somatic interventions. *Clinical Social Work Journal*, 49(4), 421-434.

(23) van der Kolk, B. A. (2005). Developmental trauma disorder: Toward a rational diagnosis for children with complex trauma histories. *Psychiatric Annals*, 35(5), 401-408.

(24) Rothschild, B. (2000). *The Body Remembers: The Psychophysiology of Trauma and Trauma Treatment*. W. W. Norton & Company.

(25) Herman, J. L. (2015). *Trauma and Recovery: The Aftermath of Violence--From Domestic Abuse to Political Terror*. Basic Books.

(26) Brave Heart, M. Y. H. (2003). The historical trauma response among natives and its relationship with substance abuse: A Lakota illustration. *Journal of Psychoactive Drugs*, 35(1), 7-13.

(27) Schore, A. N. (2003). *Affect Dysregulation and Disorders of the Self*. W. W. Norton & Company.

(28) Porges, S. W. (2004). Neuroception: A subconscious system for detecting threats and safety. *Zero to Three*, 24(5), 19-24.

(29) Earned Security Collaborative. (2013). Earned security, resolving trauma, and promoting resilience: Research to practice. *Zero to Three*, 33(4), 25-31.

(30) Schwartz, A. (2017). *The Complex PTSD Workbook: A Mind-Body Approach to Regaining Emotional Control and Becoming Whole*. Althea Press.

(31) Aposhyan, S. (2004). *Body-Mind Psychotherapy: Principles, Techniques, and Practical Applications*. W. W. Norton & Company.

www.ingramcontent.com/pod-product-compliance
Lightning Source LLC
Chambersburg PA
CBHW060508090426
42735CB00011B/2148